BASIC GUIDE TO ORTHODONTIC DENTAL NURSING

Fiona Grist

R.D.N., B.A. (Hons) OU

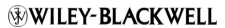

WILEY-BLACKWELL

A John Wiley & Sons, Ltd., Publication

This edition first published 2010
© 2010 Blackwell Publishing Ltd

Blackwell Publishing was acquired by John Wiley & Sons in February 2007. Blackwell's publishing programme has been merged with Wiley's global Scientific, Technical, and Medical business to form Wiley-Blackwell.

Registered office
John Wiley & Sons Ltd, The Atrium, Southern Gate, Chichester, West Sussex, PO19 8SQ, United Kingdom

Editorial offices
9600 Garsington Road, Oxford, OX4 2DQ, United Kingdom
2121 State Avenue, Ames, Iowa 50014-8300, USA

For details of our global editorial offices, for customer services and for information about how to apply for permission to reuse the copyright material in this book please see our website at www.wiley.com/wiley-blackwell.

The right of the author to be identified as the author of this work has been asserted in accordance with the UK Copyright, Designs and Patents Act 1988.

Wiley also publishes its books in a variety of electronic formats. Some content that appears in print may not be available in electronic books.

Designations used by companies to distinguish their products are often claimed as trademarks. All brand names and product names used in this book are trade names, service marks, trademarks or registered trademarks of their respective owners. The publisher is not associated with any product or vendor mentioned in this book. This publication is designed to provide accurate and authoritative information in regard to the subject matter covered. It is sold on the understanding that the publisher is not engaged in rendering professional services. If professional advice or other expert assistance is required, the services of a competent professional should be sought.

Library of Congress Cataloging-in-Publication Data

Grist, Fiona.
Basic guide to orthodontic dental nursing / Fiona Grist.
p. ; cm. — (Basic guide dentistry series)
Includes index.
ISBN 978-1-4443-3318-3 (pbk. : alk. paper) 1. Orthodontics. 2. Dental assistants. I. Title. II. Series: Basic guide to dentistry series.
[DNLM: 1. Orthodontics. 2. Dental Assistants. WU 400 G869b 2010]
RK521.G75 2010
617.6'43–dc22
2010016763

A catalogue record for this book is available from the British Library.

Set in 10/12.5 pt Sabon by Aptara® Inc., New Delhi, India
Printed and bound in Malaysia by Vivar Printing Sdn Bhd

1   2010

Basic Guide to
Orthodontic Dental Nursing

Dedication

For Michael,
with love, as always

Contents

Foreword

The role of the orthodontic surgery assistant/nurse in the delivery of orthodontic care is crucial. Every orthodontist relies on his assistant to help with the delivery of orthodontic care. The chairside is the coal-face of orthodontic delivery and the more effective and efficient this aspect of care, the better the orthodontic experience and outcome for the patient.

This book is an 'all you need to know' about assisting in orthodontic care delivery and is an invaluable learning tool and reference for all the orthodontic team. The Guide is essential reading for trainees – getting the fundamentals right early on sets a solid foundation for the day-to-day team approach.

The British Orthodontic Society (BOS), whose commitment to education is top of its activity list, welcomes and recommends Fiona Grist's *Basic Guide to Orthodontic Dental Nursing*. BOS is confident that the guide will provide invaluable instruction for the qualified orthodontic nurse, the general dental nurse and the trainee nurse.

Dr Les Joffe
CEO – British Orthodontic Society
July 2010

How to use this book

The aim of this book is to give the dental nurse in general practice an introduction to the world of orthodontics and orthodontic dental nursing. It would
also be beneficial for trainee nurses working in an orthodontic environment.

Orthodontics is a specialist branch of dentistry and has its own vocabulary.
The information in this book is a basic guide; it does not set out to:

- examine clinical features (why the problem arose)
- cover treatment planning (what is the best choice of treatment)
- treatment mechanics (how the appliances achieve what they do)

Its objectives are to illustrate what the dental nurse needs to understand to be
able to work efficiently at the chairside when treating an orthodontic patient.

There are several excellent orthodontic textbooks available if you feel you
want to develop your knowledge further. The career pathways for orthodontic
dental nurses are now wide and the possibilities are infinite. Nurses have an
important place as Dental Care Professionals in the dental team. This book
aims to be a helpful first guide on what will hopefully be a long and interesting
journey.

When reading this book different procedures for various treatments are
outlined. While it is the nurse's role to assist the clinician, there are areas that
are their sole responsibility; these are highlighted in the text in italics.

A quick glance into the stock cupboards and cabinets in an orthodontic
surgery will reveal quite different contents from that of a general dental surgery.
There will be nothing with which to fill teeth or fissure seal, no extraction
forceps or root canal trays. Anything that helps to irrigate a periodontal pocket,
whiten a tooth, prepare abutments for a bridge or fit veneers will be missing.
Cupboards in orthodontic units and practices may share the basics, such as
mirrors, probes, College tweezers, and use the same alginates and disposable
sundries, but beyond that, they have very little in common. However, these
cupboards are full, and it is not possible to cover every method or procedure,
or all materials or equipment that is in use.

Just as we had to learn what was needed for restorative, endodontic, and prosthetic procedures we need to learn what is needed for orthodontic treatment, which instruments are used for what procedure and why they are used.

Each chapter will cover a topic, with a short background and guide to what you will need to prepare so that the treatment can be undertaken as efficiently as possible. Where it seems helpful, there are photographic examples, the aim being to show the instruments as clearly as possible. The photographs are not all to the same scale.

This book does not go into detail regarding decontamination and sterilisation. The same procedures and protocols apply in orthodontics as in other specialties. The areas to watch concern the effect repeated sterilisation has on stiffening box joints on pliers. It can have a detrimental effect on pliers that have cutting edges. When sterilising pliers and instruments with beaks, always have the beaks open.

As with every skill, be it orthodontic treatment or baking a cake, everyone will have their individual method of working and their favourite tools. There is no hard and fast rule that says each procedure must be carried out using only certain instruments in the same way, in an exact order. Every clinician has their preferred methods of working and each and every nurse organises the layout of their trays, as they like them. This is as it should be, do what works best for you.

There is a saying,

You don't know what you don't know.

This book contains a lot of information but at the same time there will certainly be omissions. Every day brings new materials, new techniques and new treatment philosophies. Orthodontics is inevitably becoming split into specialties within a specialty. The pace of development and change ensures that what is current today is not tomorrow.

Hopefully, this book will achieve what it sets out to do, which is to provide enough written and visual information for a reasonable grounding of basic knowledge. Its aim is to encourage dental care professionals, especially dental nurses, to understand more about orthodontic nursing.

There is so much that as trained or trainee dental nurses you are already expert at doing, so this book will not cover knowledge you already have or skills you already possess. It is not intended to be comprehensive, rather a basic insight into the world of orthodontic nursing, it is merely a guide.

Acknowledgements

There has been no end to the tremendous support I have received from my husband Michael. He has had faith and unlimited patience. When computers, cameras, and all manner of technology were out to get me, he just quietly sorted it out. I just could not have done it without him, and I never stop telling him this.

Special thanks must go to Alan Hall who kindly gave up many, many hours of his time to look over my shoulder and check that I had not got my clinical wires crossed. Also to Maureen Dickinson who looked over my other shoulder and spent many hours checking that I did not leave out the major facts whilst busily including the minor ones. Thank you both for sharing your expertise so generously and for giving this book the benefit of your time, enthusiasm, experience and knowledge with such graciousness.

There are so many people who I want to thank. David Morris gave permission and his nurses sourced the images for use on the cover, thanks to Julie Heseldene for her phone calls. Steve Jones was kind enough to let me use his photographs of TADs. Paul Ward supplied some of his photographs of lingual appliances. Janet Goodwin at NEBDN was most helpful with permission to reproduce the Certificate of Orthodontic Nursing syllabus. Lisa McDonald at the GDC helped me with permission to use the Syllabus for Orthodontic Therapists. The Occlusal Indices are reproduced by kind permission of Professor Steve Richmond and Ortho-Care.

Orthodontics has some of the very best supply companies and I have been overwhelmed by their encouragement and willingness to help. These include Ortho-Care, DB Orthodontics, TOC, Hawley Russell, TP Orthodontics, 3M Unitek, Precision Orthodontics, Optident, Torque Orthodontics, Dental Directory and Colgate. I am grateful for their permission to use their products in the photographs.

I have had the pleasure of being associated with ONG from the beginning. You would look a long time to find harder working or more focused folk. It is impossible to mention everyone, but special thanks go to Alex Moss, Ann Jones, Denise Douglass, Debra Worthington, Janet Gray, Carly Matthews, Mary Bardet and Anne Gowans. Extra special thanks are needed for Janet Robins, a lady who leads by example and who freely shares her font of knowledge. To the many others not mentioned by name, you are not left out, you know who you are, a big thank you to you too.

My respect for the British Orthodontic Society is infinite. They have long been in the forefront in fostering the 'team' approach in orthodontics in the UK. It has been, and continues to be, hugely supportive of orthodontic nurses and they have blazed a trail for other specialties to follow. Special thanks to Ann Wright and her team, Tony, Ann, Jaki and Gavin and everyone at Bridewell Place. You set the standard.

A big thank you to my colleagues, the delightful team of folks with whom I have the pleasure of working, especially Alan Hall, Jo Clark, Angus Pringle, David Keats, Helen Signy, Judith Edwards, Peggy Taylor, Wendy Winstanley, Trudy Johns, Julia Glennon, Suzanne Ryder-Lee and Ian Bond. You make work days fun and enrich my day-to-day enjoyment of orthodontics.

Many moons ago, I received a note from Caroline Holland, asking if I would consider writing a small article about Orthodontic Nursing. While I was quite sure that I could not, it was Caroline who convinced me that I could. I owe her a huge debt of gratitude, but for her, I would not even have written the title!

Last, but by no means least, my thanks to Baljinder Kaur at Aptara and to the fantastic support team at Wiley-Blackwell, with special thanks to Katrina Hulme-Cross, Nick Morgan and Emily Jefferson, who were always there to advise and encourage, and regularly and generously went the extra mile.

Chapter 1

Definition of orthodontics and factors influencing orthodontic treatment

Orthodontics is a specialised branch of dentistry. The name comes from two Greek words:

- *orthos* – meaning straight or proper
- *odons* – meaning teeth

so the meaning is clear – 'straight teeth'.

Orthodontics is the study of the variations of the development and growth of the structures of the face, jaws and teeth, and of how they affect the occlusion (bite) of the teeth.

Ideally, there should be the same number of permanent teeth in each arch.

Any deviation from the norm is called:

- a malocclusion, if it affects teeth alignment and the bite relationship

Most malocclusions are genetically caused, i.e. they are inherited, e.g. missing teeth or a protruding mandible.

Other malocclusions can be caused by the patient, e.g. digit sucking or trauma.

Orthodontic treatment can correct a malocclusion by putting the teeth into their normal position and occlusal relationship (with surgical help, if needed) so that:

- the bite is fully functioning and the patient can bite and chew properly
- the oral hygiene is made easier, thus helping to prevent caries and gingivitis
- the malocclusion does not cause other damage
- the patient looks better and has better self-esteem

Orthodontic treatment in conjunction with orthognathic (maxillo-facial) surgery can correct an underlying jaw discrepancy or facial asymmetry.

DEFINITION OF ORTHODONTICS

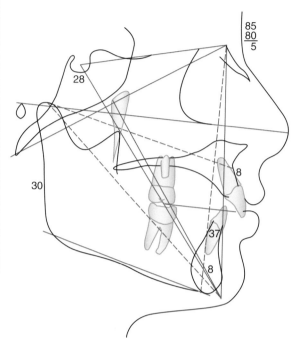

Figure 1.1 Cephalometric tracing.

Orthodontic planning is done in conjunction with the surgeons using clinical and radiographic assessment, with a cephalometric tracing (Figure 1.1) often analysed using computer software program.

So, orthodontists set out to:

- straighten teeth
- improve the bite
- improve the function
- improve oral hygiene (and make teeth easier to clean)
- improve self-esteem of the patient

CLASSIFICATION OF OCCLUSION

When assessing occlusion there are two aspects to classification:

- incisor relationship
- buccal segment occlusion, left and right

Both are recorded on a patient's Orthodontic Assessment Form.

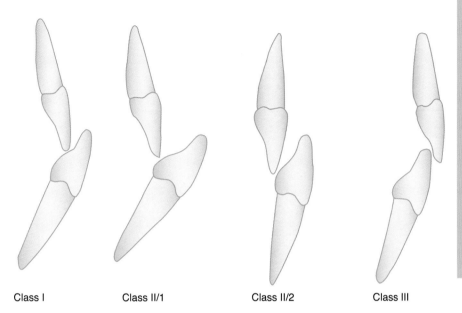

Class I   Class II/1   Class II/2   Class III

Figure 1.2 Incisor classification.

Incisor classification

- Classes have roman numerals, e.g. I, II, III
- Divisions do not, e.g. Class II/1 or Class II/2

The incisor classification (Figure 1.2):

- relates to the bite of the tip of the lower central incisors onto the back of the upper central incisors
- is divided into three horizontal sections and where the lower incisor occludes will determine the classification

Class I
- The incisal edge of the lower incisors bites on or below the cingulum plateau of the upper incisors

Class II/1
- The upper incisors are proclined or upright (Figures 1.3 and 1.4)
- The lower incisors bite behind the cingulum plateau of the upper incisors
- The position of these front teeth means they can be damaged more easily because of their vulnerable position

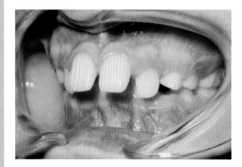

Figure 1.3 Large overjet.

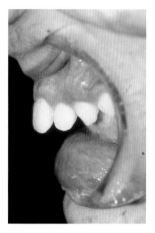

Figure 1.4 Side view of severe overjet.

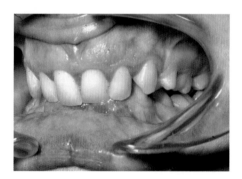

Figure 1.5 Bite stripping lower gingivae.

Class II/2

- The upper incisors are retroclined
- The lower incisors bite behind the cingulum plateau
- The position of the teeth can, when closed, lead to trauma to the lower labial gingivae and the upper palatal gingivae (Figures 1.5–1.7)

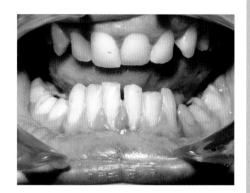

Figure 1.6 Damage to labial gingivae caused by bite.

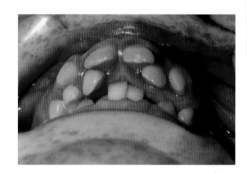

Figure 1.7 Bite causing trauma to the palate.

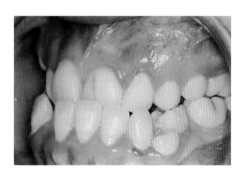

Figure 1.8 Class III.

Class III

- The bite is edge to edge or reversed
- The incisal edge of the upper incisors can bite into the back (lingual) surface of the lower incisor (Figure 1.8)
- A horizontal overlap is called **overjet**
- A vertical overlap is called **overbite**

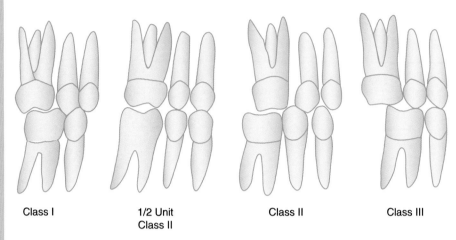

Class I   1/2 Unit   Class II   Class III
                            Class II

Figure 1.9 Diagram of buccal segment occlusion.

Buccal segment occlusion

The buccal segment occlusion (Figure 1.9):

- was devised by Edward Angle in 1890
- is still widely used today
- is based on the occlusion between the first permanent molar teeth, which erupt when the patient is about 6 years old

There are three classes:

- **Class I** – This is as near to the correct relationship as you see
- **Class II** – This is at least half a cusp width behind the ideal relationship
- **Class III** – This is at least half a cusp width in front of the ideal relationship

THE MIXED DENTITION

Sometimes parents see their child's perfectly straight deciduous (baby) teeth fall out only to be replaced by a 'jumble' of crowded permanent teeth (Figure 1.10).

A combination of full-sized teeth in a face that still has a lot of growing to do often prompts parents to request an early orthodontic opinion. Permanent teeth can look huge in little faces.

The average times for permanent tooth eruption are:

- Age 6
  - 1/1 lower central incisors
  - 6/6 lower first molars
  - 6/6 upper first molars

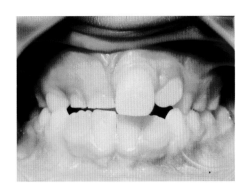

Figure 1.10 Mixed dentition.

- Age 7
  - 1/1 upper central incisors
  - 2/2 lower lateral incisors
- Age 8
  - 2/2 upper lateral incisors
- Age 11
  - 3/3 lower canines (cuspids)
  - 4/4 lower first premolars (bicuspids)
  - 4/4 upper first premolars (bicuspids)
- Age 12
  - 3/3 upper canines (cuspids)
  - 5/5 lower second premolars (bicuspids)
  - 5/5 upper second premolars (bicuspids)
  - 7/7 upper second molars
  - 7/7 lower second molars
- Age 18–25
  - 8/8 upper third molars (wisdom teeth)
  - 8/8 lower third molars (wisdom teeth)

Normally, patients begin orthodontic treatment between 10 and 13 years of age. At 10–11 years, they are still in the mixed dentition with:

- some deciduous teeth
- some permanent teeth
- some teeth yet to erupt

INDICATIONS FOR TREATMENT

Clinical indications for orthodontic treatment may be because the teeth:

- are overcrowded
- may have erupted out of position

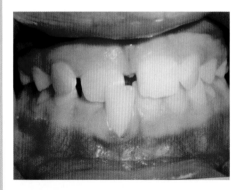

Figure 1.11 Lower incisor trapped outside the bite.

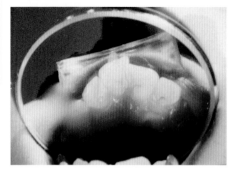

Figure 1.12 Caries between overlapping teeth.

- are protruding – Class II/1
- are in a reverse bite
- are in a self-damaging bite (Figure 1.11)
- are spaced
- are absent – hypodontia
- are damaged

Where there is a mild malocclusion, i.e.:

- with only very small irregularities
- where the tooth position does not compromise oral hygiene
- which does not interfere with function, e.g. biting off food, eating

orthodontic treatment may not be indicated, as it may not be seen to significantly improve dental health.

Those cases, e.g.:

- with overcrowded, protruding teeth
- with rotated teeth which make oral hygiene difficult and cause problems with caries (Figure 1.12)
- which visually deviate from average, e.g. a reverse bite
- which look unattractive and affect the smile
- which seriously affect function, e.g. makes chewing food difficult

are classed as malocclusions warranting treatment.

UNDERLYING CAUSES OF MALOCCLUSION OF THE TEETH

There may also be:

- underlying skeletal abnormalities
- facial asymmetries

These can be:

- hereditary (run in families, e.g. tendency to be Class III)
- a result of injury
- a result of illness affecting facial or skeletal growth
- a result of a syndrome or cleft

These may require orthodontic treatment as part of a multi-disciplinary care treatment pathway.

MULTI-DISCIPLINARY APPROACH

Some patients require orthodontic treatment in conjunction with other dental specialties.
  These include:

- restorative (e.g. hypodontia patients needing implants/bridges or microdontia patients needing veneers or crowns)
- surgical (e.g. patients needing an osteotomy)
- cleft (e.g. patients needing alveolar bone grafting)

These patients have their orthodontic treatment in coordination with the other specialties.

Problems when the arch is not intact

One of the aims of orthodontic treatment is to have each tooth in its correct place within the dental arch.
  If a tooth is malaligned (out of its correct position), it is not necessarily an isolated problem; it has a domino effect.
  The teeth on either side of it may also be out of their correct position and the opposing tooth does not have the correct occlusion (bite).
  If there is no tooth to oppose it, a tooth may supra-erupt. Contact points are lost, teeth rotate and, because they are no longer self-cleansing, food traps are created, where fibres can get lodged or packed.
  As a consequence of this, plaque is encouraged to accumulate:

- which inflames the gingivae (gums)
- which encourages periodontal pockets

In the young patient this is not too drastic, as it probably has not yet become a significant issue.

In adult patients, however, following orthodontic treatment, it may be necessary to restore incisal edges or fill cervical abrasion cavities, which only become apparent when the teeth have been corrected.

BRUXISM

- Young patients, towards the end of the deciduous dentition, can often present with teeth almost ground down to gingival level. It may continue into the mixed dentition and is often quite noisy and noticeable when it occurs in sleep
- For some older patients with severe bruxism, an occlusal guard can be made to be worn overnight during sleep. This attempts to limit the damage that is done to the incisal and occlusal surfaces of the teeth
- Anxious patients also grind and clench their teeth during the day when under stress

DIGIT SUCKING

Some patients continue to suck their fingers or thumbs well beyond the age when their deciduous teeth have been replaced by their permanent successors. A prolonged habit is one which exists beyond the age of 7 years.

It may adversely affect the bite and position of the anterior teeth and can produce a unilateral buccal crossbite, an asymmetrical anterior open bite (where the digit enters the mouth) (Figure 1.13) or an increased overjet. How much damage is caused depends on for how long the thumb or finger is sucked and how strong the habit is.

These patients may try really hard to break this habit.

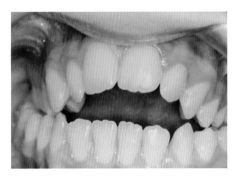

Figure 1.13 Anterior open bite due to digit sucking.

It is possible to fit a removable upper anti-habit appliance, which is worn full-time or sometimes when they are asleep.

It is an upper removable appliance that has prongs in the centre of the palate, which act as a positive deterrent for the thumb or finger. This usually breaks the habit.

DENTAL HEALTH

Some problems are caused by:

- diet – too much sugary or acidic food or drink (dental caries)
- tooth brushing – the wrong technique, too hard a brush
- acid reflux – symptom of bulimia
- medication – side effect of some medication inhalers

Damage to teeth resulting in tooth surface loss comes under the general headings of:

- Attrition – bruxists (patients that grind their teeth, often during sleep)
- Abrasion – excessive wear, e.g. overenthusiastic tooth brushing
- Erosion – acid attack on the enamel, found in fresh fruit juice, diet drinks and stomach acids (reflux in eating disorders)
- Abfraction – a tooth being 'high on the bite' and being overloaded

CONDITION OF THE SURROUNDING SOFT TISSUES

Lips

Lips can be:

- competent – when they are at rest they come together easily and form a good oral seal
- incompetent – when at rest they do not close, or if they are closed, the lips are strained, often as a result of posturing. This closure is only temporary

Tongue

- The tongue works with the lower lip to form a seal when swallowing
- A tongue which tends to thrust can push forward and 'splay' the front teeth out

The position of the teeth and the form of the dental arches are determined by the balance of the soft tissues between tongue and lips/cheeks.

Chapter 2

The first appointment

Orthodontic patients are usually referred by their own dentist (their general dental practitioner (GDP)) for specialist orthodontic treatment.

These referrals can be sent to:

- an orthodontic specialist practitioner
- a community orthodontist
- a consultant orthodontist
- a dental practitioner with special interest (DPwSI) and some basic training in orthodontics

Some adult patients may choose to self-refer.

The referring dentist may wish to send the patient to an orthodontist to:

- see and advise
  - if there are teeth that are slow to erupt
  - if there are teeth that have submerged
  - if there are teeth that are in a self-damaging position
- see and monitor
  - if the patient is dentally too young for treatment
  - if there are already signs of adverse dental development, i.e. growth, facial asymmetry or crowding
- see and treat
  - if the second dentition has developed but is overcrowded
  - if there is a complex problem
  - if there is a multi-disciplinary need

The referral letter needs to contain as much relevant information for the orthodontic practitioner as possible.

Apart from the basic data:

- name
- address
- telephone numbers (land, mobile, work, etc.)
- date of birth
- National Health number
- name of general practitioner (doctor)

it also needs to give:

- clinical reason for referral (what the dentist feels is the problem)
- medical history (if it is helpful to know in advance, e.g. attention deficit hyperactivity disorder, autism, deafness or dental phobia)
- dental history (good oral hygiene, high caries level, etc.)
- any previous orthodontic history (e.g. previous assessment or treatment)
- social history (e.g. supportive family, regular check-ups)
- what the patient/parent is concerned about ('fangs', teasing)
- whether the patient is concerned at all (quite happy to stay as they are)
- likely compliance (supportive family, patient keen)

When the referral letter is received, the patient (or their parent or guardian if they are underage) is sent an appointment.

On the first visit, a full orthodontic assessment is carried out (Figures 2.1 and 2.2).

This includes:

- checking the name and age of the patient
- finding out what is of concern to the patient
- full medical history, including whether the patient
  - has allergies (nickel, latex, etc.)
  - is currently under the care of a doctor for any reason
  - has had any operations
  - is taking medication of any kind
  - has asthma, if so, type of inhalers
  - has diabetes
  - has or had chest or heart conditions

Patients and/or parents are asked to fill in and sign a health questionnaire form. This is updated and checked regularly.

It includes details of:

- school or college (day or boarding)
- work
- contact sports played
- musical instruments played by mouth
- any digit (thumb or finger) sucking, bruxism (tooth grinding)

THE CLINICAL ASSESSMENT RECORDS

These begin with extra-oral features and then move on to intra-oral ones.

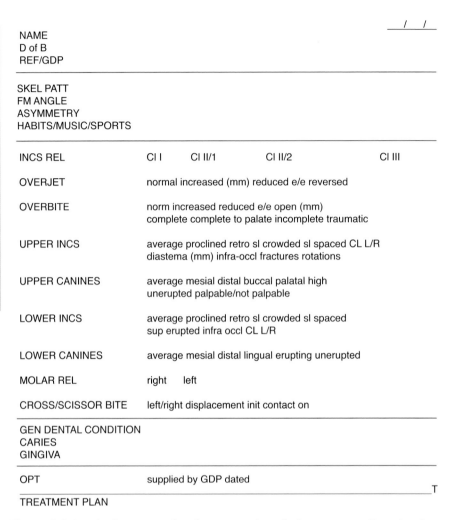

_____ / _____ /

NAME
D of B
REF/GDP

SKEL PATT
FM ANGLE
ASYMMETRY
HABITS/MUSIC/SPORTS

INCS REL	CI I	CI II/1	CI II/2	CI III
OVERJET	normal increased (mm) reduced e/e reversed			
OVERBITE	norm increased reduced e/e open (mm) complete complete to palate incomplete traumatic			
UPPER INCS	average proclined retro sl crowded sl spaced CL L/R diastema (mm) infra-occl fractures rotations			
UPPER CANINES	average mesial distal buccal palatal high unerupted palpable/not palpable			
LOWER INCS	average proclined retro sl crowded sl spaced sup erupted infra occl CL L/R			
LOWER CANINES	average mesial distal lingual erupting unerupted			
MOLAR REL	right left			
CROSS/SCISSOR BITE	left/right displacement init contact on			

GEN DENTAL CONDITION
CARIES
GINGIVA

OPT   supplied by GDP dated
                                                                                    T
TREATMENT PLAN

Figure 2.1 Sample of assessment form from a specialist orthodontic practice. (Reproduced with the kind permission of Alan Hall, South Downs Orthodontic Practice.)

Skeletal pattern

The maxilla-to-mandible relation in the antero-posterior plane:

- Class I
- Class II
- Class III
  - mild
  - moderate
  - severe

ORTHODONTIC CONSULTATION -

Patient Details Age: years months	Medical History	Dental History

Complaint	Social Details

Skeletal Pattern

AP 1 2 3	Vertical ↑ ↓ Average	Lateral Asymmetry Yes No

Soft Tissue Pattern

Lips Competent Incompetent	Lip Line High Low Average	Habit Yes No

Teeth Present	Missing Teeth

Tooth Quality	Oral Hygiene	Caries/Decalcification
Good Fair Poor	Good Fair Poor	

Lower Labial Segment

	Mild Mod Severe	Mild Mod Severe		
Aligned	Crowded	Spaced	Proclined Retroclined Average	CL L R Centre

Upper Labial Segment

	Mild Mod Severe	Mild Mod Severe		
Aligned	Crowded	Spaced	Proclined Retroclined Average	CL L R Centre

Lower Buccal Segments	Aligned Crowded Spaced
Upper Buccal Segments	Aligned Crowded Spaced

In Occlusion	OJ ↑ ↓ Average mm
	OB ↑ ↓ Average Complete Incomplete

Molar Relationship Right	I II III $\frac{1}{4}$ $\frac{1}{2}$ $\frac{3}{4}$ 1
Molar Relationship Left	I II III $\frac{1}{4}$ $\frac{1}{2}$ $\frac{3}{4}$ 1
Incisor Relationship	I II/1 II/2 III
Crossbites Yes No	Displacement Yes No

Figure 2.2 Sample of assessment form from a hospital orthodontic department. (Reproduced with the kind permission of Jo Clark, Worthing and Southlands Hospitals NHS Trust.)

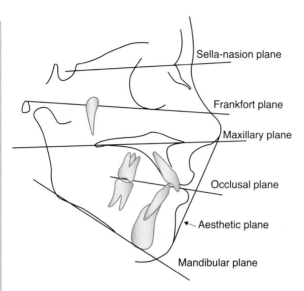

Sella-nasion plane

Frankfort plane

Maxillary plane

Occlusal plane

Aesthetic plane

Mandibular plane

Figure 2.3 Drawing showing relation of FM angle.

FM (Frankfort-mandibular) angle (Figure 2.3)

- high
- average
- low

Asymmetry

- This is usually mandibular

Soft tissues

- Lips
  - line
  - competency
  - expressive behaviour
  - if lower lip is behind upper incisors
    (This is the end of the extra-oral examination.)
- Tongue
  - size
  - position in mouth
  - swallowing behaviour
- Tonsils
  - if there is a history of difficulties in breathing through the nose, snoring or repeated sore throats

- Frenum
  - upper
  - lower

Gingivae and oral hygiene

- health of the gums
- presence of plaque

Charting of the teeth

- present
- absent (unerupted or extracted)
- presence of caries/restorations/fissure sealant
- erosion
- enamel hypomineralisation
- hypoplasia
- size discrepancy, e.g.:
  - microdont, small tooth (microdontia)
  - megadont, large tooth (megadontia)
- supernumeraries – teeth which are additional to the norm:
  - most often found in the anterior maxilla
  - can be conical or tuberculate

Incisor relationship (Figure 2.4a)

- Class I
- Class II/1
- Class II/2
- Class III

Overjet

Horizontal measurement between upper and lower incisors:

- normal (3 mm)
- increased (record the measurement in millimetres)
- edge to edge
- reversed

Overbite

- upper incisors overlap

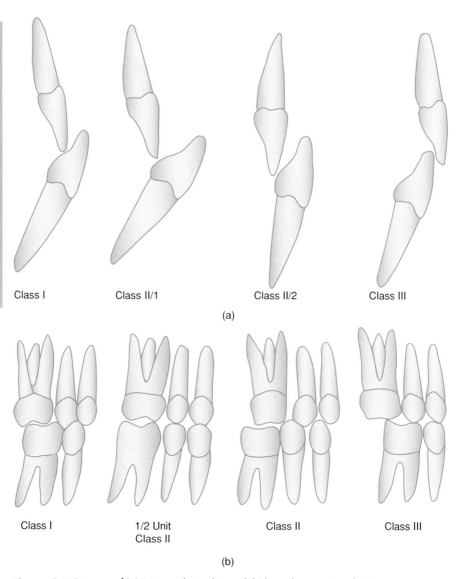

Class I   Class II/1   Class II/2   Class III

(a)

Class I   1/2 Unit   Class II   Class III
                 Class II

(b)

Figure 2.4 Diagram of (a) incisor relationship and (b) buccal segment occlusion.

- lowers in vertical plane
  - normal (3 to 4mm)
  - increased
  - reduced
  - edge to edge
  - open (record the measurement in millimetres)
  - complete
  - complete to palate

- incomplete
- traumatic

Upper and lower incisors

- average inclination
- proclined
- retroclined
- crowded
- rotations
- spaced
- diastema (record space in millimetres)
- centre line
- infra-occluded
- supra-erupted
- any fractures/restorations
- any abnormal mobility
- mesial or distal inclination
- buccal or palatal/lingual

Upper canines

- average inclination
- high
- unerupted but palpable
- unerupted but not palpable
- mesial or distal
- buccal or palatal

Lower canines

- average inclination
- mesial
- distal
- buccal
- lingual
- erupting
- unerupted

Molar relationship (buccal segment occlusion) (Figure 2.4b)

- Class 1
- 1/2 unit Class II

- Class II
- Class III

Crossbite

- localised
- unilateral (arch widths do not match one side)
- bilateral (arch widths do not match both sides)

Scissor bite

- lingual crossbite of lower teeth

Open bite

- anterior
- posterior
- lateral

Displacement of mandible when closing

- left
- right
- anterior
- initial contacts

NB: This distinguishes the term from displacement of teeth in the Index of Orthodontic Treatment Nee (IOTN).

Note must also be made of any:

- submergence (teeth that have 'sunk' down back into the gum)
- impactions
- damaged teeth (e.g. repaired/unrepaired, root filled or ankylosed)
- poor-quality, long-term, outlook teeth (e.g. heavily filled or hypoplastic)
- transpositions (teeth in exchanged positions, e.g. a canine mesial to a lateral)
- other anomalies

There is a 'benchmark' to achieving the ideal occlusion known as the six Andrews' keys.

These are:

- Class I molars
- correct incisor inclination
- correct tip
- no spaces
- no rotations
- flat curve of Spee

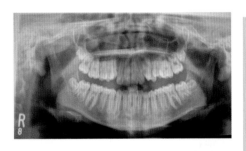

Figure 2.5 Example of OPT radiograph.

RADIOGRAPHS

If the orthodontist wants to further assess the patient, then radiographs are needed. These are an invaluable diagnostic tool when formulating a treatment plan.

The two formats most routinely used in orthodontic assessment are:

1. The orthopantomogram (OPT) (Figure 2.5)
   - is an extra-oral radiograph
   - is a panoramic view of both the maxilla and the mandible
   - shows all the underlying skeletal structures, including:
     - temporo-mandibular joints (TMJs)
     - position of the condyles (head of the rami)
     - level of bone (in some older patients there can be bone loss)
     - sinuses
     - position of dental nerve canals, e.g. inferior dental nerve
     - any cysts
     - radiolucencies
   - also shows the dental features:
     - position of the teeth
     - any unerupted or impacted teeth
     - any ectopic teeth (teeth that have developed and erupted, or not erupted, in their correct position)
     - supernumerary teeth
     - any anomalies of the teeth, e.g. fusing of roots
     - the presence of third molars (wisdom teeth)
     - the condition of any teeth that may have cavities or deep restorations (these may influence any decision on the possible need for extractions)

NB: OPTs are not taken to show caries, but often do. Bite wing radiographs are needed if there is concern regarding cavities.

2. The lateral cephalometric radiograph (Figure 2.6):
   - is an extra-oral radiograph
   - shows a true lateral (side) image of the skull and face

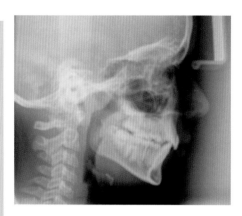

Figure 2.6 Example of cephalometric radiograph.

- shows angulation of incisor teeth
- is used to monitor skeletal growth, e.g. if the mandible is developing adverse forward growth (Class III)
- is used if there needs to be tracings made for measurements in proposed surgical planning

Other radiographs used for diagnosis and treatment in orthodontics include:

- upper occlusals (used if the OPT is not clear in the upper incisor region)
- upper lateral occlusals
- periapicals
- postero-anterior skull

The use of cone beam computed tomography is becoming more widespread for orthodontic use.

There is also the possibility to take three-dimensional radiographs known as computed axial tomography scans. Computed axial tomography scans can assist in producing computer-aided design/computer-aided manufacturing models of the skull, maxilla and mandible, and three-dimensional facial soft tissue scans.

These radiographs can involve a greater amount of radiation than the other types used.

Following clinical assessment and using the OPT and lateral skull radiograph if required, the orthodontist can then formulate the treatment plan.

It is important to establish why the patient is seeking treatment, as this will influence their keenness and compliance.

- Are they themselves motivated (they want it for themselves)?
- Are they being told they need it (they are trying to please someone else)?

With the radiographs in hand, the orthodontist can then ask the patient and parent if they have any questions.

These may include:

- what is the aim of the orthodontic treatment?
- how it is to be achieved?
- what does the treatment involve?
- when is the best time for this to be done?
- is it better to do the treatment in stages?
- once started, how long will it take?
- how many weeks between the appointments?
- will extractions be needed as part of the treatment?
- which appliance (brace) or sequence of appliances will be needed?
- will treatment hurt?
- what type of retention will be needed and for how long will it need to be worn?
- will it still be possible to play sport; can a mouth guard be worn with a brace?
- will it be possible to continue to play musical instruments by mouth, e.g. flute, saxophone, trumpet?

The clinician may want to take photographic records.
These usually follow:

- a set position of each view required both intra- and extra-orally
- the same camera and background
- the same angles

so that there is standardisation of all the images taken.

Some clinicians have access to a photographer, some take the photographs themselves and many nurses are excellent photographers.

RISKS OF ORTHODONTIC TREATMENT

When assessing treatment options and the benefits that treatment will bring, the orthodontist also advises the patient and parent of any possible risks that might occur. These risk factors can occur in a minority of cases and some can easily be avoided (Figure 2.7).

Decalcification

- Patients with poor oral hygiene can develop inflamed and unhealthy gums and may not be accepted for treatment
- Patients that do not comply with oral hygiene instructions may experience decalcification/caries as a result of poor brushing, eating sweets and drinking

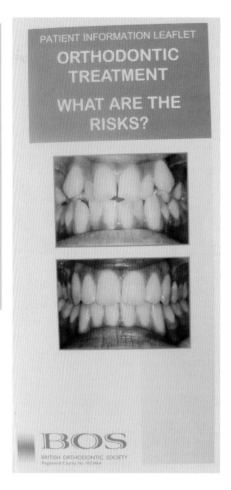

Figure 2.7 Leaflet on risks of orthodontic treatment.

fizzy drinks. The end result can be damaged teeth. In these cases, the use of fluoride mouthwashes, toothpastes gels, and mousse must also be encouraged
- Failure to comply with oral hygiene may result in the early termination of treatment

Resorption

- Sometimes, there is a need to take end-of-treatment radiographs, these may show that there has been slight shortening of the roots on some teeth. This resorption happens during tooth movement. It is monitored and is rarely of significance, but the patient and their dentist need to be aware if it is significant for future dental reference

Relapse

- Adverse tooth movements after completion of orthodontic treatment – This can be caused by adverse growth or failure to comply with retainer wear

Patient dissatisfaction

- The patient feels that the aims and objectives set out at the discussion of treatment were, in their opinion, not met

DISCUSSION AND CONSENT

Patients often have lots of questions and the orthodontic nurse is often the person they ask. It is at this time that the relationship starts to build between them. The nurse will get to know the patient over the course of the many visits and various procedures, and a friendly, relaxed relationship will help to encourage their motivation and compliance. It is important that the patients enjoy contributing to and feeling part of their orthodontic journey as much as possible.

After the assessment and treatment-planning discussion when an agreement has been reached and they consent to proceed with treatment, baseline records will be taken. Like radiographs, these are:

- legal documents
- helpful in diagnosis and treatment planning
- needed for monitoring and scoring occlusal indices
- needed for case presentations

Under English Law, if the patient is under 16 years, the legal age of consent, their parent or guardian must give informed consent. However, if the patient has a full understanding of the proposed procedure, they can consent themselves even if they are under the age of consent.

TAKING BASELINE RECORDS

Information leaflets may be given at this stage to take home and read.

On the first appointment for treatment, the nurse needs to prepare:

- *the patient's clinical notes*
- *mouth mirror*
- *probe*

THE FIRST APPOINTMENT

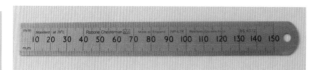

Figure 2.8 Orthodontic ruler.

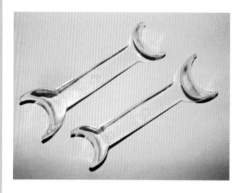

Figure 2.9 Lip retractors.

- *orthodontic ruler (Figure 2.8)*
- *hand mirror*
- *alginate, bowls and a spatula (putty (vinyl polysiloxane) can be used, but less likely when taking study models)*
- *impression trays*
- *wax (and bite registration recorder if used)*
- *wax knife*
- *method of softening wax, e.g. flame, blow torch, hot water*
- *glass of mouthwash and tissues*
- *laboratory sheet with instructions for technician*
- *solution to disinfect impressions*
- *camera (ring flash and digital)*
- *lip retractors (Figure 2.9)*
- *photographic mouth mirrors (Figure 2.10), if to be used*
- *information leaflets for the patient*
- *oral hygiene instruction leaflet for the patient*

For the chairside procedure, the nurse:

- *ensures that the staff and patient are wearing personal protection*
- *ensures that the patient is seated comfortably in the chair*
- ensures that a wax squash bite is taken to record the occlusion
- ensures that upper and lower alginate impressions are taken
- *ensures that after disinfection, both impressions and bite are taken to the technician with instructions*

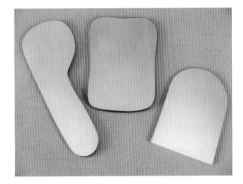

Figure 2.10 Photographic mouth mirrors.

- *takes/assists with taking the photographs using lip and cheek retractors and/or mouth mirrors*

Views include:

- intra-oral
  - left lateral
  - centric
  - right lateral
  - profile or lateral incisor view
- extra-oral
  - full face, smiling
  - full face, not smiling
  - 3/4 view
  - profile, not smiling

The patient is given a leaflet on proposed treatment.

Any further questions are answered.

It is ensured that the patient has the correct series of appointments booked in.

Patients benefit from being given:

- a leaflet on their proposed treatment
- a leaflet on oral hygiene

If they are given these at this appointment it gives them an opportunity to spend some time reading them before their next 'fitting' appointment. They can then get an idea of what will be happening when they attend for the start-of-appliance treatment.

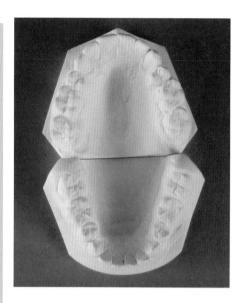

Figure 2.11 Example of trimmed orthodontic models.

ORTHODONTIC MODELS

When back from the technician, the study models must be boxed and a record made of the identification number and where they can be found.

This is recorded:

- in the model-boxing book which is kept in the model box store
- in the patient's notes

(See Chapter 23 on model box storage.)

NB: Orthodontic study models are reproductions of the dental arches and how they occlude together as they were on the day that they were taken, and must always be marked with the patient's name and date when taken.

They are trimmed in a specific way, known as Angle's trimming (Figure 2.11).

The upper model base does not have a rounded front. It is 'pointed' and angled.

The lower model does have a rounded front.

Also, when the upper and lower models are trimmed together with the wax bite between them, it should be possible to:

- lay them on their side or 'heels' (i.e. with the front teeth facing upward) on a flat surface
- pick them up in the same position in which they were put down
- make them stand without rocking and the teeth should stay together in the correct occlusion

PHOTOGRAPHS

The photographs taken must be recorded in the photographic log book.

Increasingly, many images are digital and stored on computer but need to be backed up securely.

However, if they are hard copy, they must be filed either in the patient's notes or in the hanging photograph files.

Photographs and radiographs are part of the patient's records. Clinical governance and good practice require that they must be stored securely to comply with current legislation concerning data protection.

Depending on the treatment plan, the patient is now ready:

- for the active treatment to begin and an appliance to be fitted

or

- to begin a period of monitoring and watchful waiting, sometimes when there is a need to monitor adverse growth

THE FIRST APPOINTMENT

Chapter 3
Occlusal indices

The demand for orthodontic treatment has grown steadily over the years. The public's awareness of the condition of their teeth and smile has driven the desire to have 'straight teeth' and a confident smile.

As a result of this, more and more patients are asking to be referred to an orthodontist for treatment.

The Index of Orthodontic Treatment Need (IOTN) was devised as a scale for standardising measurement, by including:

- degree of severity
- aesthetics

The increasing demand for treatment may mean that not all patients that would like treatment are eligible to receive it under a third party funded system, e.g. the National Health Service (NHS).

Where there are finite resources, there has to be a balance between what is wanted and what is needed. This means a prioritising of treatment and takes into account:

- the entry levels for treatment
- the availability of funds and clinician
- the hierarchy of treatment providers

To assess the needs of a patient using a standard set of criteria means that each orthodontic assessment arrives at a similar conclusion.

As such, it needs to have several functions.

- It needs to be an assessment that uses a series of 'benchmark criteria'
- It needs to measure the severity of the presenting conditions
- It needs to assess whether by treating their orthodontic problem the patient would have significant benefits

IOTN has two components.

DENTAL HEALTH COMPONENT

This is to measure and quantify the severity of the malocclusion in the categories, which range from IOTN 5, which is the most severe, to IOTN 1, which measures no significant deviation from normal (Figure 3.1).

In any malocclusion, the one presenting the worst deviation from the norm is measured.

These may include:

- supernumerary teeth
- impacted teeth
- a reverse overjet
- displacement of teeth
- severe rotations
- crossbites
- hypodontia (missing teeth)
- an increased overjet

The Dental Health ruler is helpful in maintaining a consistent method of taking measurements (Figures 3.3 and 3.4). It prioritises in descending order:

- M – missing teeth
- O – overjet
- C – crossbite
- D – displaced contact points
- O – open/overbite

AESTHETIC COMPONENT

This shows the appearance of the teeth – what the patient looks like. It is used in conjunction with scoring of 3 on the dental health component.

It is a sheet showing 10 photographs of increasing severity of malocclusion.

These are all the same size, are produced in colour and are anterior views of the teeth in occlusion (Figure 3.2).

They range from:

- 1 – which has no irregularities, an acceptable occlusion

to

- 10 – which has severe irregularities where the malocclusion is in greater need of treatment

The patient is asked which photograph looks most like their teeth.

OCCLUSAL INDICES

TABLE 1   THE DENTAL HEALTH COMPONENT
          OF THE INDEX OF ORTHODONTIC TREATMENT NEED (IOTN)

GRADE 5 (Need treatment)

5.i Impeded eruption of teeth (except for third molars) due to crowding, displacement, the presence of supernumerary teeth, retained deciduous teeth and any pathological cause.

5.h Extensive hypodontia with restorative implications (more than 1 tooth missing in any quadrant) requiring pre-restorative orthodontics.

5.a Increased overjet greater than 9mm.

5.m Reverse overjet greater than 3.5min with reported masticatory and speech difficulties.

5.p Defects of cleft lip and palate and other craniofacial anomalies.

5.s Submerged deciduous teeth.

GRADE 4 (Need treatment)

4.h Less extensive hypodontia requiring prerestorative orthodontics or orthodontic space closure to obviate the need for a prosthesis.

4.a Increased overjet greater than 6mm but less than or equal to 9mm.

4.b Reverse overjet greater than 3.5mm with no masticatory or speech difficulties.

4.m Reverse overjet greater than 1mm but less than 3.5mm with recorded masticatory and speech difficulties.

4.c Anterior or posterior crossbites with greater than 2mm discrepancy between retruded contact position and intercuspal position.

4.1 Posterior lingual crossbite with no functional occlusal contact in one or both buccal segments.

4.d Severe contact point displacements greater than 4mm.

4.e Extreme lateral or anterior open bites greater than 4mm.

4.f Increased and complete overbite with gingival or palatal trauma.

4.t Partially erupted teeth, tipped and impacted against adjacent teeth.

4.x Presence of supernumery teeth.

GRADE 3 (Borderline need)

3.a Increased overjet greater than 3.5mm but less than or equal to 6mm. with incompetent lips.

3.b Reverse overjet greater than 1mm but less than or equal to 3.5mm.

3.c Anterior or posterior crossbites with greater than 1mm but less than or equal to 2mm discrepancy between retruded contact position and intercuspal position.

3.d Contact point displacements greater than 2mm but less than or equal to 4mm.

3.e Lateral or anterior open bite greater than 2mm but less than or equal to 4mm.

3.f Deep overbite complete on gingival or palatal tissues but no trauma.

GRADE 2 (Little)

2.a Increased overjet greater than 3.5mm but less than or equal to 6mm with competent lips.

2.b Reverse overjet greater than 0mm but less than or equal to 1mm.

2.c Anterior or posterior crossbite with less than or equal to 1mm discrepancy between retruded contact position and intercuspal position.

2.d Contact point displacements greater than 1mm but less than or equal to 2mm.

2.e Anterior or posterior openbite greater than 1mm but less than or equal to 2mm

2.f Increased overbite greater than or equal 3.5mm without gingival contact.

2.g Pre-normal or post-normal occlusions with no other anomalies (includes up to half a unit discrepancy).

GRADE 1 (None)

1.   Extremely minor maloccusions including contact point displacements less than 1mm.

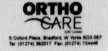

ORTHO
CARE
5 Oxford Place, Bradford, W Yorks BD3 0EF
Tel (01274) 362017 Fax (01274) 734446

Figure 3.1 Dental Health Component. (Reproduced by kind permission of Ortho-Care.)

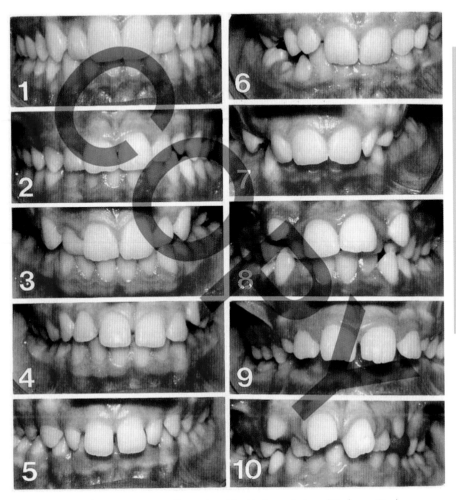

Figure 3.2 Aesthetic Component. (Reproduced by kind permission of Professor Stephen Richmond and Ortho-Care.)

PAR

This stands for the Peer Assessment Rating and is used to assess the effectiveness of treatment and the improvement it has achieved, using the before and after study models.

Many clinicians also use these findings for audit purposes.

There are small clear rulers (Figures 3.3 and 3.4) for measuring the occlusal features on study models, with scoring sheets to record the score on pre- and post-treatment models to gauge the level of effectiveness. This is recorded as greatly improved, moderately improved or little or no improvement.

OCCLUSAL INDICES

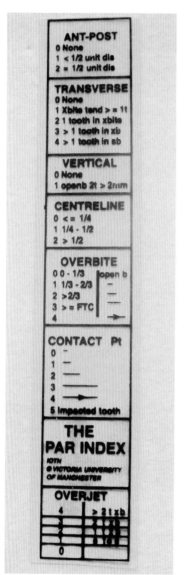

Figure 3.3 PAR Index ruler (disposable).

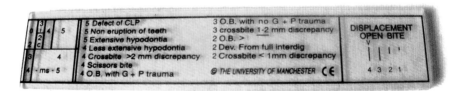

Figure 3.4 PAR Index ruler (autoclavable).

ICON

This stands for Index of Complexity, Outcome and Need. It is a development from IOTN and also includes the complexity of treatment.

MANAGEMENT

Under the NHS, the referrals may go through their local Managed Clinical Network and are allocated to the clinicians by the local Primary Care Trust/Organisation. These are sent to either:

- primary care – the specialist orthodontic practices

or

- secondary care – the hospital services

At the present time to receive funding in:

- primary care, the patient needs to have an IOTN rating of 3.6 or above to qualify
- secondary care, the patient needs to have a score of 4 or 5

The Primary Care Trusts have an appeals procedure for dealing with cases whose score puts them in the low priority category.

If their assessment is borderline or the patient, parent or clinician feels that they merit inclusion for treatment, their case can be sent to the Review Panel for Patients with Individual Needs (PIN) to ask them to adjudicate.

If the PIN panel decides that the patient does not qualify, the parent can accept this or fund the cost of treatment themselves.

The IOTN ensures that the same criteria are universally used.

Note: The scan scale was first published in 1987 by the European Orthodontic Society (Ruth Evans and William Shaw, For rating dental attractiveness. European Journal of Orthodontics 1987;9:314–318).

Chapter 4

Motivation

In general, patients who are undergoing orthodontic treatment are quite enthusiastic about their treatment.

Maintaining this enthusiasm can be difficult but it truly is the secret of success.

Orthodontic treatment involving fixed appliance therapy takes:

- 18–24 months on average
- regular visits

and the optimum time to do this is in the early second dentition.

For a young patient, perception of time is quite unlike that of their orthodontist or parents. They are brought up in a world of no-waiting, touch-of-a-button, on-demand instant results.

Most patients see a school term as a long period and the time between one birthday and the next is off the scale. So, when they start treatment that is probably the keenest they are going to be.

Orthodontic treatment is like planting a garden; you plant and wait patiently until the flowers appear and you sometimes have a long period before you can see any signs of progress.

Sometimes, in the early stages when the 'instant fix' that patients hope for is just not happening, they become despondent when they look at themselves and see little progress.

When we reach this stage, there are often telltale signs:

- oral hygiene can deteriorate
- there are breakages
- there are occasional missed appointments
- the patient can become uncommunicative, even sullen

This is where the motivation has to be rekindled.

Unlike patients in general practice, orthodontic patients:

- are referred in from their regular dentist
- are seen for a course of treatment and retention
- are not routinely seen again

During orthodontic treatment, patients are seen, on average, every 4–6 weeks.

During that, time you get to know them and their parents quite well.

Sometimes they may have had a brother or sister in treatment before them so that both the parents and new patient will be familiar with the surgery and the routine of appliance adjustment appointments.

Many have friends at school who are undergoing the same treatment and may be having similar experiences to cope with.

This can be helpful, if it is constructive.

Not being the only one with a brace helps.

There is much discussion of treatments between patients, especially at school. Like all chatter:

- there are those who tell tales of doom and gloom
- there are others who tease
- on rare occasions, banter may become bullying

If this happens, parents and schools must get involved. It must be stopped.

When orthodontic patients are assessed, the amount of support they will get is important.

The range of scenarios includes:

- a keen patient with a keen and supportive parent
- a keen patient with an indifferent or unsupportive parent. We can get a result, but it is hard work
- a patient who is actively against treatment with a parent who insists they must have it

(These parents want their child to receive treatment and the child has to comply. This may be because the parent wants what they see as the best for their child, maybe they missed having the treatment themselves or failed to complete it and always regretted it.)

As these reluctant patients look you right in the eye with the:

- 'just you see who is the boss'
- 'I really, really don't want this'
- 'I will have the last word'

look, it is the beginning of an uphill struggle, often littered with many breakages and lost appliances along the way!

When the nurse builds a rapport with a patient it is easier to know what motivates them.

As the treatment progresses, the patient experiences a mixture of:

- *seeing the benefits appearing*
- *wanting the braces removed as soon as possible*

There needs to be a steady stream of encouragement at this stage.

Often, for the younger patient, visual encouragement in the form of a sticker helps. It is surprising what the power of a sticker can achieve!

MOTIVATION

Keep reinforcing and encouraging the positives such as:

- *how good the teeth are looking*
- *show them the start models, 'look how far we have come already!'*
- *remind them what they looked like before treatment*
- *emphasise how much of the hard work is already done*
- *try to have a provisional deband date to aim for, e.g. off before the school prom or before they go on holiday*
- *keep praising the positive and cajole on all the negative areas*

The best motivation comes from the patients themselves, but if they hear you say:

- **'you are doing SO well, what a star', the smile you get tells you that together you will get there**

If the oral hygiene is in the doldrums:

- *show photographs of results that poor cleaning might bring*
- *give them a new type of interspace brush*
- *give them a couple of tubes of different toothpastes*

If they are wearing elastomerics (O-rings), encourage them to make their own choice of colours to try and give them back ownership of the appliance, pride in their efforts and achievement in undergoing the therapy.

At the deband appointment, admire, admire and admire again!

Nature helps us here, as most teenage patients present with:

- malaligned, often protruding teeth
- many problems associated with hormonal teenagers

However, by the deband date, there are huge improvements on all fronts and the 'ugly duckling' patient who began treatment has been transformed into a confident swan.

There is nothing to compare with the look of absolute delight when the sometimes-awkward, rebellious, monosyllabic teenager of a couple of years ago looks in the mirror and sees the changes. You have come to know them, their highs and lows, what music they listen to, their sports, their clothes, what is going on in their lives and sometimes their anxieties and concerns. It is quite amazing just how much you do get to know about them.

Their treatment is like a journey you have travelled together. As a nurse, you have helped when their enthusiasm flagged and when the temptation to eat everything that is banned overtook them; so you are part of their success. A great result for them is a great result for you too. For orthodontic nurses, this special relationship with the patient you know for such a short time is one of the main differences between nursing in orthodontics and general practice.

MOTIVATION

However, it is not all over yet:

- with the malocclusion corrected
- the teeth aligned

we are about to enter the retention phase!

RETENTION

The majority of patients wear their retainers as and when asked and have no problems.

For a few patients the feeling is that:

- they have finished treatment
- their braces have been removed
- there are no more monthly appointments to keep

with straight teeth, their mission is accomplished.

Patients are always told that teeth after debanding can (and will!) move if the retainers are not worn. However, a few patients think that this is something that happens to other people. They decide when and how to wear their retainers hoping that it will probably be enough to get them through.

Alas not.

It may not be a matter of 'will the teeth move' but 'how far will they go'.

Relapse is disappointing for everyone involved.

Retention is probably one of the hardest stages with which to get the patient to comply.

They may have reacted well to compliance whilst in active treatment because they were regularly encouraged and reminded.

Motivation is not the same. You can get a patient who is not self-motivated to comply; they just do what is asked of them. Once you are out of sight and for them, out of mind, it is then down to the patient to encourage themselves, to be self-motivating and regulate themselves.

These patients often develop a very relaxed attitude to wearing their retainers!

For whatever reason, some patients will return to the surgery many months, often years, after their braces were removed with teeth a long way from the way they were on the day they were debanded.

Nine times out of ten, away from regular visits to the surgery, the motivation to wear the retainers was no match for the:

- 'I'll risk it, it will be OK!' hopefuls

Some are lucky and get away with it; many more are not.

MOTIVATION

So, at the retainer fitting appointment:

- *tell your patients how great they look*
- *compare their teeth now with their initial models and photographs*
- *warn them that Nature will fight back, given half the chance*
- *empower them to follow the regime for wearing their retainers*
- *tell them it is really important*
- *tell them not to risk undoing all the hard work they, and everyone else, have put in and keep on enjoying the great smile they have now got*

PATIENTS WHO READILY COMPLY

Sometimes adults come in for treatment (see also Chapter 21).

Their needs may vary:

- from correcting mild overcrowding
- to completely rehabilitating that patient's occlusion

Whatever their malocclusion may be, it is a concern to them. For these patients especially, the improvement to their appearance, and often function, will boost their self-esteem.

Some patients have lived with and been unhappy with their problem for a long time. These patients have a great deal of compliance and self-motivation.

The orthodontic team

However, while patient motivation is vital, of equal importance is the motivation of the individual members of the orthodontic team.

Motivated staff perform well. They are:

- proactive
- happy in their work
- positive
- efficient

In short, they are empowered.

Orthodontists have long acknowledged their nursing staff to be 'key' members of a highly specialised and productive team. Every individual within the team has a role to play and each member of the team recognises their reliance on each other. Once established, trust within a team ensures valuable cooperation to, if and when the need arises, solve problems and resolve issues.

Accepting and sharing responsibility is a powerful motivator when team members are empowered.

- It reflects in their work
- They become more productive
- They are excellent ambassadors for their practice/department/unit

Motivation in the team setting can come from:

- above

the clinicians who
- involve and encourage their nurses to learn more
- delegate responsibilities
- develop their potential
- provide Continuing Professional Development (CPD)
- sideways

colleagues
- other nurses in the surgeries
- reception and clerical staff, managers
- technicians
- colleagues you meet at conferences or meetings
- people who get you interested in what new things they are doing
- networking
- below
  - nurses that have just started working in your work place and need your training and encouragement
  - nurses that are learning new techniques and need demonstrations to give them an extra skill
  - nurses that you are mentoring who need support

- Motivation is enthusiasm
- Empowerment fuels enthusiasm
- Enthusiasm develops the individual

If you are motivated yourself, you lead by example.

When they are motivating their patients,
Orthodontic nurses don't just 'Talk the talk', they 'Walk the walk'

Chapter 5

Leaflets

Orthodontic treatment is complex and the patient needs to play their part in looking after and adjusting their appliances where necessary.

For a patient and their parent an important part of being able to comply with what is being asked of them, is to fully understand:

- exactly what it is that they need to do
- why they are doing it
- what they are aiming to achieve

In order to do that, there must be good communication between the patients and the clinician.

Therefore, we need to:

- create trust between the orthodontic team and the patient
- persuade and influence them to carry out the instructions
- impress on them their role in getting the best result at the end of treatment

Leaflets given to the patient should cover two areas:

- information – what the treatment entails, what the patient can expect, etc.
- instruction – their contribution to the treatment, what they need to do, etc.

There are many leaflets available and the orthodontic nurse needs to select the most appropriate one for each situation.

The British Orthodontic Society produces many excellent leaflets on matters of clinical guidance (Figure 5.1).

These include:

- advice on digit/dummy sucking
- orthodontic management of the medically compromised patient
- advice on the use of headgear and face bows
- use and storage of digital photographs
- orthodontic records – collection and management

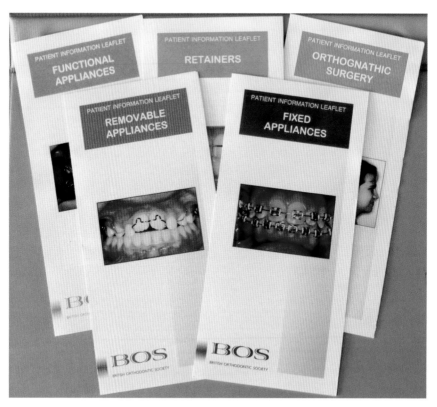

Figure 5.1 BOS information leaflets. (Reproduced with the kind permission of the British Orthodontic Society.)

These are some of the many leaflets that are printed on a wide and diverse range of subjects. They are useful for the orthodontic nurse to read and to update on current best practice.

The most commonly used leaflets are the ones that you give to patients.

When verbal instructions are given to a patient it is often:

- at the end of a procedure which has been tiring for them
- when they may be anxious
- when they may feel stressed about how strange the appliance feels
- when they and their parents are glad having an appliance fitting is over and are not fully listening to what is being said
- at a time when they and their parents are worried about a specific concern, e.g. needing to have teeth extracted

Often, they do not fully listen to what is being said; they are just listening for and focused on any aspect of concern to them. In many cases, it may be the words 'extraction' or 'headgear'.

When trying to get information across to patients it has been estimated that:

- only 7% of communication is verbal
- 38% is passed on by the speed and tone of voice
- the main part, a massive 55% of the message, is delivered visually

What the patient sees, be it body language or eye contact, engages the patient's attention. The patient might remember how they felt when you spoke to them but they do not always recall what you said. Anxiety is a barrier to listening and understanding.

So, with this in mind, after the patient has been given advice and instructions verbally by the nurse, it is really beneficial that they are given a printed instruction leaflet as well. This can be read later.

They take this home and can refer to it when they are not under any pressure and can take the information in more effectively. Given that the majority of patients are young, it is also better to repeat information that they may have forgotten than to assume that they know, remember and understand it, than end up with a problem.

When the patient has their new patient consultation appointment sent out to them, it is helpful to enclose a 'First Visit to the Orthodontist' leaflet (Figure 5.2).

This just outlines what is likely to happen, what will be discussed, etc. For many patients, the thought of this visit is quite worrying, and some children who have not had any experience of dental treatment, e.g. fillings, do not know what to expect. Often, their peers at school take advantage of this anxiety and make them quite anxious. Some patients even worry that when treatment starts their teeth will be taken out there and then!

If the patient knows what is likely to happen, they may not be totally relaxed but the reassuring information in the leaflet goes a long way to helping them get a good night's sleep, and to be able to eat their breakfast before they arrive in the chair. This makes them more receptive to listening and understanding what is being said.

Also, leaflets are given at the beginning of each phase of treatment.

- They always reinforce the messages
- They tell the patient the aims of treatment
- They tell the patient how it will affect them
- They tell the patient what type of braces they will need to have
- They tell the patient how to best cope with them
- They tell the patient how to look after and clean them

In addition, the leaflets can have the names of the nurses they will meet when they have their first appointment and during any treatment. This can foster a more personal relationship.

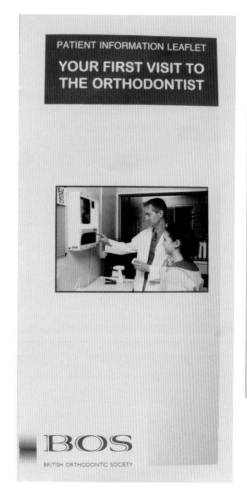

Figure 5.2 'First visit to the orthodontist' leaflet. (Reproduced with the kind permission of the British Orthodontic Society.)

The leaflets also provide contact numbers, thereby encouraging the patient to feel that should there be anything about which they are unsure, a quick phone call to the surgery for clarification will be better than worrying unnecessarily.

Sometimes patients find the prospect of orthodontic therapy daunting and they can become anxious. Another explanation and a little empathy can usually dispel this. *The nurse can often pass on to the orthodontist any area which is particularly worrying a patient. The nurse can act as the facilitator, often broaching a subject or asking a question on the patient's behalf. In this way, patients, or their parents, will feel able to mention concerns that they think are silly or minor, but which are causing genuine anxiety.*

Good leaflets are in colour with informative, easy-to-understand text and clear photographic images. If there is any apprehension concerning treatment, it is often helpful to give the patient the leaflet before they start treatment.

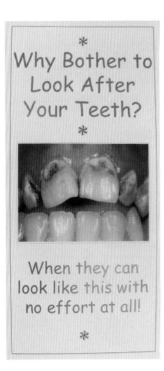

LEAFLETS

Figure 5.3 Leaflet in a different style. (Reproduced with the kind permission of the Ortho-Care.)

In this way, they can get used to the idea and 'get their heads round it' so that it is not an unknown entity. It is the patients with the "unknown" to deal with that their friends find so easy to scare.

There are very many styles and types of leaflets available.

Clinical subjects covered include:

- fixed appliances
- removable appliances
- functional appliances
- extra-oral traction
- retainers
- mini screws
- oral hygiene

While some are produced by professional bodies, e.g. British Orthodontic Society, others are commercially produced to enhance or endorse a product. These are produced in a different style (Figure 5.3).

Many practices and individuals design and produce their own leaflet. These are often created 'in-house' as a combined effort from all staff of a practice or department.

'In-house' leaflets can be really helpful if they include extra information that covers emergency details, e.g. what they need to do if they have a problem. This information includes details of who to contact, the emergency telephone numbers, etc. This can be reassuring for patients and leaflets containing such information are often stored at home in a safe place 'just in case'.

Sometimes, empowering a patient gets good results, e.g. if they need to keep a diary or log of their participation in treatment. You are, in effect, asking them to provide information about themselves. You are not reinforcing what they need to do, they are affirming that they know what to do.

Asking them to keep a 'food diary', a sticker progress chart or to 'trial' which type of interspace brush or toothpaste they find most effective can make them proactive. For some patients, this focuses them and they take ownership of the actions.

For younger patients, never underestimate the power of a sticker, this is a 'travelling leaflet', a written endorsement of how well you think they are doing.

LEAFLETS

Chapter 6
Oral hygiene

The majority of patients wearing orthodontic appliances are teenagers and as a group they are always hungry and need regular intakes of food. They tend to snack between meals and very often the wise words on the dietary sheet given to them in the surgery when their appliance is fitted is forgotten or ignored. When the tummy rumbles between meals or temptation, in the form of a hard, sticky or crunchy snack, is put in their path. Either way, the wise words on the advice sheet fly from their thoughts as the food flies into their mouths.

The oral hygiene leaflet should be a way of helping the patients to help themselves, to maximise all the effort they put in by doing the right things in the right order.

If they do this, they minimise the danger of permanently damaging their teeth by decalcification and decay.

So, how effective is an oral hygiene leaflet and how do you, as a dental nurse, get your patient to take the advice on board?

FOR REMOVABLE APPLIANCES

Removable braces have acrylic baseplates which can trap food between them and:

- the palate
- the lips
- the tongue

Patients are advised after every meal (and snack!) to:

- remove the appliance and clean it under running water, using regular toothpaste
- do this over a sink which is full of water; should the appliance slip out of the patient's hand, it will not shatter on the basin
- clean their teeth thoroughly
- clean their palate and gums, taking extra care around the gum margins
- once a week, soak the appliance in a cleaner, such as Retainer Brite (Figure 6.1), which is designed especially for the purpose

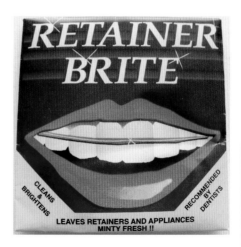

Figure 6.1 For removable appliance cleaning.

No appliance can be self-cleansing and trapped food debris can irritate the soft tissues of the mouth and they can become inflamed.

FOR FIXED APPLIANCES

Fixed appliances are not the easiest to keep clean, but the consequences of not doing so are permanently marked or decayed teeth.

Straight but marked teeth is not a good look. Try and impress on patients that these are *their* teeth they are damaging. It is their responsibility!

Besides regular tooth brushing, and flossing if possible, the orthodontic patient has to be extra careful with:

- hard, sticky or crunchy foods
- sweets or crisps between meals
- fizzy or cola drinks
- chewing gum
- fresh fruit juice (especially if drunk between meals)

The problems and consequences are as follows:

- Sucking sweets, such as mints and toffees, leads to cervical decalcification
- Eating hard, sticky or crunchy foods damages brackets, clasps and archwires
- Fresh fruit juice, diet and 'cola' type drinks are acidic, attacking the enamel on the tooth surface, making the tooth surface glass-like, especially if 'swished' around teeth. This can erode the incisal edges and may lead to sensitivity (drinking straight from a can could make this worse); will attack the plaque trap areas around brackets and wires (Figure 6.2)
- Chewing gum can get stuck around wires and brackets

ORAL HYGIENE

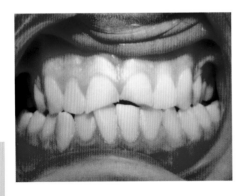

Figure 6.2 Incisal erosion due to fizzy drinks drunk from a can.

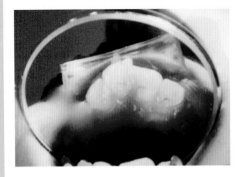

Figure 6.3 Caries between overlapping teeth.

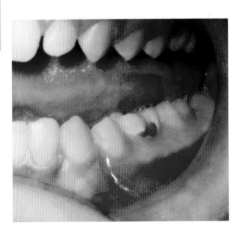

Figure 6.4 Cervical caries.

- Mints can be sucked slowly, often held in the buccal sulcus (They can have a high sugar content which is leached into the saliva and into the plaque, which turns to acid, which leads to caries; Figures 6.3 and 6.4.)

Figures 6.3 to 6.5 are not the images of their teeth that patients are expecting.

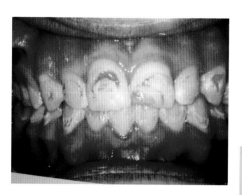

Figure 6.5 Decalcification of teeth after deband.

Show them photographs of the damage (Figure 6.5), warning them, *'is it worth the risk'?*

WAYS PATIENTS CAN HELP THEMSELVES TO PREVENT PROBLEMS

Toothbrushes and brushing

It does not really matter whether patients use a manual or an electric brush; it is what they do with it while it is in their mouths that counts. However, a brush with a small head is very helpful and some electric brushes now have small heads especially designed for orthodontic use.

Patients need to have a routine, a sequence of brushing so that every part of the mouth gets cleaned and nothing gets overlooked.

They also need to know for how long to brush and to use a timer if it helps them.

Do not use the same brush until it is almost bald; change it regularly.

It is advisable to clean thoroughly after breakfast and also before bedtime so that the mouth is clean overnight.

If it is not possible to use a toothbrush when they are out or at school during the lunch break, a vigorous rinse with water to dislodge the worst of the debris is better than nothing. But a travel brush is better! These need to be washed and dried out overnight, out of their protective cover.

Toothpaste

It is advisable for patients to use toothpaste which contains fluoride.

ORAL HYGIENE

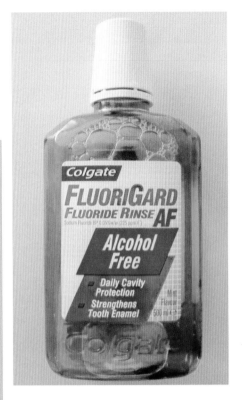

Figure 6.6 Fluoride mouth rinse.

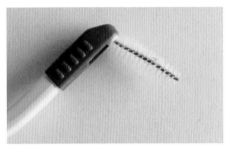

Figure 6.7 Interdental brush.

Fluoride mouth rinse

During and after treatment, a fluoride mouth rinse (Figure 6.6) is recommended.

Interdental brushes

Food debris from biscuits and crisps can be soft and is easily trapped around the brackets and wires of fixed appliances or around the gingival margins of removable appliances where it adds to the build-up of plaque.

It is important that patients use interdental brushes (Figure 6.7).

Floss

Floss is not easy for younger patients to use. Getting it wound around the fingers and inserting it over and under arch wires takes manual dexterity, is a learned skill and is very time-consuming.

Some floss:

- is now flavoured which is popular with the patients
- has a fluoride coating which is popular with the orthodontists

Disclosing tablets

Patients are encouraged to check that their standard of plaque removal is up to speed by using a disclosing tablet about once a week (Figure 6.8). This can be demonstrated to them at the chairside and then after that they can do it for themselves at home. Fixed appliances especially are full of little plaque traps and *must* be cleaned effectively.

Disclosing tablets are made from vegetable dye. They are usually coloured red or blue with the tablets being more popular and convenient. It is helpful to check that patients do not have intolerance to Erythrosine, E number 127, as it is used in some tablets.

(It is advisable to warn patients not to use these tablets just before they are going out, as it will stain the lips. A blue tinge to the lips can be a bit alarming as can a bright red tongue!)

After a routine brushing, the patient either chews a tablet or rinses with disclosing solution for a minute. They then spit out any that is left in their mouth and look in the mirror. The plaque that is left on the teeth will be stained (Figure 6.9). The patient needs to then go back and clean their teeth again, this time being aware of the areas that they are missing out.

ORAL HYGIENE

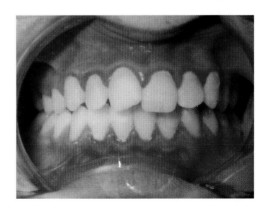

Figure 6.8 Effect of plaque on teeth.

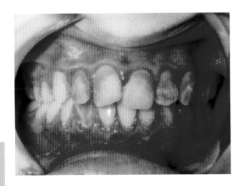

Figure 6.9 Disclosing tablets showing plaque.

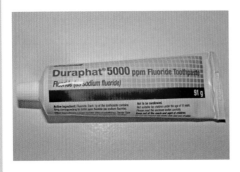

Figure 6.10 Fluoride toothpaste.

Tooth mousse

At the completion of fixed appliance treatment, some clinicians like to encourage their older patients to:

- use a toothpaste that has a higher level of fluoride content
- use tooth mousse, which is a water-based, sugar-free, topical cream

Tooth mousse contains calcium and phosphate but not fluoride.
Tooth mousse helps to:

- reduce sensitivity
- neutralise pH values in the saliva
- restore lost minerals
- strengthen dentine and enamel

Fluoride toothpaste (Figure 6.10) containing increased amounts of fluoride (as sodium fluoride) up to 5000 ppm (parts per million) is now available.
Both these will help to reverse the effects of decalcification and to remineralise teeth.

Dietary advice

Rather than focus on what the patient cannot have, try and be positive and tell them what they can have and when is the best time to have it.

- Chocolate is acceptable, if:
  - it is broken into very small pieces and is not eaten straight from the fridge
  - it is eaten with a meal and is then followed by tooth brushing
- Raw carrots, apples and crusty bread can also be cut into tiny, bite-sized mouthfuls rather than trying to bite into them
- Diluted fruit juice can be enjoyed once a day with breakfast

Banning all the foods they like encourages patients to break the rules.
So,

a little leeway helps the feel good factor
which helps the compliance
which fuels the motivation
which moves the brush!

ORAL HYGIENE

GETTING THE MESSAGE ACROSS

Patients and their parents are always given oral hygiene leaflets (Figure 6.11), for advice and instructions at each phase of their treatment.

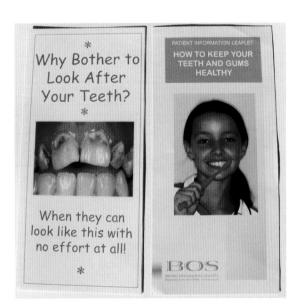

Figure 6.11 Two different styles of leaflet. (Reproduced with the kind permission of Ortho-Care and of the British Orthodontic Society.)

Most patients comply with the rules and they fully appreciate that it will only be for a relatively short length of time and that it will be in their own best interest in the long term.

They understand that there is no point having lovely straight teeth if the overall effect is marred by:

- enamel that is marked
- cavities, especially in the front teeth
- gum recession
- decalcification
- erosion

When the warnings fall on deaf ears

Patients who are not keeping their mouths healthy are warned that orthodontic treatment will be terminated early if the oral hygiene is falling below the expected standard.

This is not a hollow threat; in extreme cases, it does happen and appliances are removed before the end of treatment.

Sometimes, patients who do not heed warnings and are facing the termination of treatment:

- ask that they be given another chance
- are sorry when they realise that the appliances are being removed
- may have resigned themselves to living with irregular teeth
- often, if the patient promises to try harder the treatment is continued with a view to debanding as soon as a reasonable result has been achieved.

The long-term damage to dental health caused by poor oral hygiene outweighs the benefits of orthodontic treatment.

Poor oral hygiene is one of the most common reasons why some patients who are eligible for, and would benefit from, orthodontic treatment do not receive it.

Nurse's role

Unlike most treatments, there is no clinical procedure to follow and no instruments to prepare.

There are many ways to deliver the message.

- *The orthodontist may give the oral hygiene instruction*
- *The nurse may do it*
- *It may be a combined effort*

If there were issues around poor cleaning before the patient was accepted for treatment, and it was an area of concern which had to be improved prior to

ORAL HYGIENE

treatment being considered, you will have to be more aware and the patient will have to try extra hard to achieve the required standard.

SUPPORT

It is always useful to remember that some patients do not get the same level of parental help and encouragement as others.

While some patients may have parents that buy them every brush and mouth rinse they need, there are other patients who come from homes where dental care generally does not have a high priority and they get little or no support.

This makes some patients' job harder, and that makes the nurse's role harder too.

THE UNENTHUSIASTIC PATIENT

However, there are patients who are less than keen to undertake any orthodontic treatment at all, for whatever reason.

They are extremely anti and are not keen to even be in the surgery.

For whatever reason, their parent or parents are equally adamant that they should receive it.

They are on a collision course.

The parents are often well intentioned.

They themselves may have not been given the opportunity or did not complete their own treatment when young and they regret this and don't want their child to do the same.

They are insisting for very good reasons and they 'encourage' or press their child into it.

Often, poor oral hygiene is the only way that these 'voiceless' patients can register their protest.

It is sometimes possible to tempt this small cohort of patients by explaining that the treatment will progress much quicker if the mouth is clean.

If these patients start orthodontic treatment they, the clinician and the nurse are on an uphill struggle; they often want the appliances off early!

Basically, you just have to try to keep them communicating with you.

THE NURSE'S ROLE

The nurse is the person who should monitor oral hygiene and:

- *give encouragement when it is falling below standard*
- *praise when it is good*

ORAL HYGIENE

When a patient is doing well:

- *tell them*

It is motivating just being told you are doing something positive and doing it well.

    On the other hand, if the standard is low:

- *it is very demotivating to hear only negative comments, even though they might be true, so try and also highlight what they are doing well*

Some nurses make their own oral hygiene literature and handouts.

    Often, they compile a set of photographs to show patients when they are describing what their teeth might look like if they, and the appliances, are neglected.

    The oral hygiene regime that these patients are learning now, will hopefully be the one that takes them all the way through life and ensures that they will have good dental health and need never lose their lovely straight teeth.

ORAL HYGIENE

Chapter 7

Removable appliances

Teeth move as a reaction to forces applied to them.

There are two main types of orthodontic appliance:

- removable
- fixed

Sometimes a fixed or removable appliance can have similar aims, for example:

- a fixed appliance for maxillary expansion
- a removable appliance with a central widening screw in the midline for expansion (Figures 7.1 and 7.2)

Some treatments can be completed by using only removable appliances.

Removable appliances are sometimes used prior to a fixed appliance.

Patients will often incorrectly refer to an active removable appliance as a 'retainer'.

At the completion of any active treatment, there is a period of retention for which retainers are made. Occasionally, if treatment is with removable appliances, these can be made passive to act as retainers.

Retainers are passive appliances and maintain the position of the teeth after treatment.

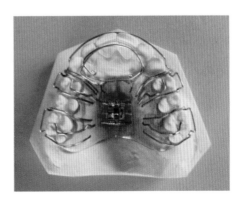

Figure 7.1 Removable appliance with expansion screw.

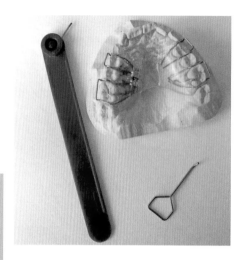

Figure 7.2 Expansion screw and choice of key types.

Removable appliances can move teeth using labial bows, screws, springs and elastics, and have been very popular in the UK, but following the development of fixed appliance therapy they have become less used.

The functional appliance is usually a removable appliance in as far as it can be taken in and out, but has different aims of treatment and is discussed in Chapter 11.

Removable appliances move teeth by tipping or tilting them whilst fixed appliances have the ability to move teeth bodily (crown and root) without tipping.

Removable appliances can be used:

• in the maxilla
• in the mandible
• both in the maxilla and in the mandible at the same time

but are more often used in the upper arch.

They are mostly used for the treatment of simple malocclusions or for short periods of time as part of an overall plan.

They are most commonly used:

• as an anterior bite plane (to reduce an increased overbite)
• to move incisors over the bite (usually in the mixed dentition)
• to tip teeth labially, lingually, mesially or distally
• to provide freeway space to correct an occlusal problem (disengage the occlusion)
• to widen an arch to correct a crossbite by using inbuilt expansion screws

Like any other appliance, they sometimes need to be repaired. In the case of removable appliances, this means the appliance has to be taken from the patient and sent to the laboratory. The breakage may be severe enough to make the appliance irreparable such that it is simpler for the technician to make a new appliance.

Removable appliances can be used in conjunction with the extraction of teeth.

This provides space into which teeth can be moved in order to reduce crowding.

To be successful, removable appliances must:

- be worn full time as instructed
- be worn by a keen patient
- be fitted in a clean mouth

In addition to removable appliances with active components which are used to move teeth, they are also used as:

- anti-habit appliances (these appliances are used to deter digit sucking)
- stimulation plates to encourage eruption, where a pad of acrylic presses over an eruption site, to encourage a late erupting tooth to appear
- space maintainers – worn to prevent teeth drifting
- retainers

The components are:

- A – anchorage
- R – retention
- A – active
- B – baseplate

The removable appliance needs to have:

- retention (to make sure the appliance is held in place), e.g. clasps/cribs
- parts to move the teeth, e.g. springs or screws
- a baseplate that fits around the teeth securely and carries all the metal components and also provides anchorage

ADVANTAGES – WHAT THEIR BENEFITS ARE

They:

- are, for an experienced technician, simple to make
- are easy to wear (for children)
- can reduce an overbite
- can tilt teeth
- need very little chairside time to fit

- make oral hygiene easier by being removable
- are less visible

DISADVANTAGES – WHAT THEY CANNOT ACHIEVE

- cannot de-rotate teeth
- cannot move the root bodily, can only tilt the position of a tooth
- can be taken out and not worn

PARTS OF A REMOVABLE APPLIANCE

Baseplate

- made of acrylic
- provides stability (anchorage) for those teeth not being moved
- carries all the active springs, screws and wires that will put force on teeth
- carries all the retention components, e.g. clasps/cribs

Often, the baseplate (Figure 7.3) can include the following.

Bite plane
This can be either:

- **Anterior**
    - acrylic build-up behind the upper front teeth to 'jack open' the bite so that the overbite can be reduced. Because the lower teeth bite onto plastic, it disengages the bite and allows eruption of buccal segment teeth

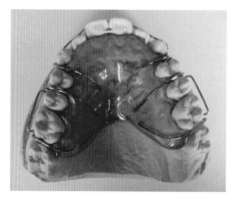

Figure 7.3 Baseplate.

- **Posterior**
  To include overlays over the back teeth to allow movement where there is
  - need to correct crossbites
  - an increase of overbite – Temporarily reducing the overbite allows upper incisor(s) to be moved 'over the bite' in Class III cases

Anchorage

Anchorage is a point from which force is delivered.
  It is achieved by:

- making the acrylic baseplate fit around palatal or lingual surfaces and includes teeth other than those being actively moved
- using baseplate together with clasps for retention of appliance
- using the slope of the palatal vault, e.g. when retracting upper canines and incisors

The active components

These are the parts of the appliance that exert force, one end of which is embedded in the acrylic base and the other against the surface of the tooth being moved.

- Springs
  - cantilever
  - Roberts retractor
  - finger
  - Z (Figure 7.4) and T springs
- Clasps
  - Adams (Figure 7.5)
  - Southend (Figure 7.6)

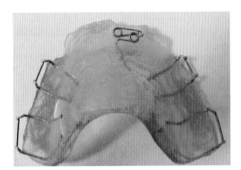

Figure 7.4 Removable appliance with Z spring.

REMOVABLE APPLIANCES

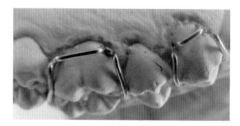

Figure 7.5 Adams clasp (crib).

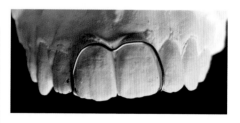

Figure 7.6 Southend clasp.

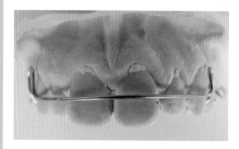

Figure 7.7 Labial bow.

- Bows
  - labial (Figure 7.7)
- Screws
  - expansion
- Elastics
  - can be attached from some of the metal components

MAKING, FITTING AND ADJUSTMENT

The fitting and adjustment of removable appliances needs removable appliance pliers, acrylic burs and a handpiece for trimming.

There is a great variety of choice in pliers and hand instruments and clinicians will have their individual preferences.

There are a number of suggested ones as named in a guide for the nurse's role, but they are unlikely to be used all at the same time.

For the chairside procedure, the nurse needs to prepare the following.

For the first appointment, the nurse needs to prepare:

- *personal protective equipment for the patient and staff*
- *alginate powder, liquid and liquid measure*
- *putty (vinyl polysiloxane) if preferred*
- *upper and lower impression trays*
- *bowl and spatula*
- *receiver in case of gagging reflex*
- *sheet wax*
- *heat source for wax*
- *wax knife*
- *disposable cup of mouthwash*
- *tissues*
- *laboratory sheet*
- *disinfectant solution for impressions*
- *sealable plastic bags, named and dated*
- *leaflet about removable appliances (Figure 7.8)*

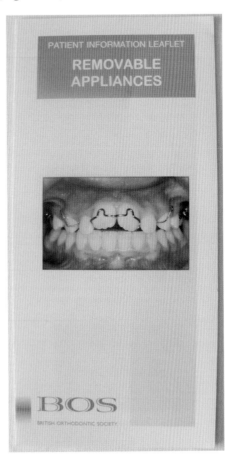

Figure 7.8 BOS Leaflet. (Reproduced with the kind permission of the British Orthodontic Society.)

REMOVABLE APPLIANCES

Procedure:

- *Ensure that the dentist, nurse and patient wear personal protective equipment*
- *Sit patient in the upright position for comfort when taking impressions*
- *Provide the patient with a bib, disposable cup of mouthwash and tissues*
- *Select upper and lower trays*
- *Extend trays with ribbon wax if needed*
- *Prepare softened wax bite; this is in a 'horseshoe shape', two sheets of wax thick*
- *The bite registration will then be taken*
- *Mix alginate or putty (lower impression usually taken before the upper)*
- *Disinfect the alginate impressions and the wax bite*
- *Give clinician laboratory card to fill in design, etc.*
- *Add the date and time of next appointment*
- *Discuss again the treatment plan and the brace with the patient*
- *Answer any questions and check that the patient understands the explanatory leaflet*

The disinfected impressions and wax bite then go to the technician. They are cast to make:

- working model for the appliance
- study models

Note that orthodontic models are trimmed in a specific way (Figure 7.9).
The models will be named and dated when they return from the laboratory.

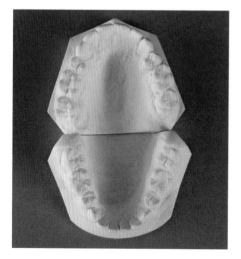

Figure 7.9 Example of the method of trimming orthodontic models.

REMOVABLE APPLIANCES

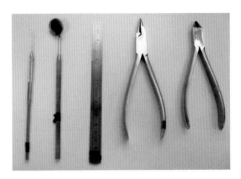

Figure 7.10 Removable appliance tray.

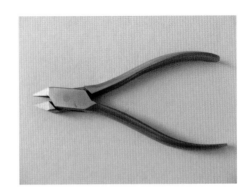

Figure 7.11 Close-up of Adams pliers.

This must be checked before they are filed into the patient's model box. It is useful to have a protocol in the practice or unit on how this is done. Having the date on the front of the models is helpful.

At the fitting appointment, the nurse needs to prepare:

- *clinical notes*
- *the appliance*
- *a tray containing (Figure 7.10)*
  - *a mirror*
  - *a probe*
  - *Adams pliers (Figure 7.11)*
  - *spring forming pliers*
  - *a ruler*
  - *dividers (optional)*

Also, there must be within reach:

- *Mauns heavy wire cutters*
- *screw key (if patient has an expansion plate)*
- *handpiece and acrylic burs*

REMOVABLE APPLIANCES

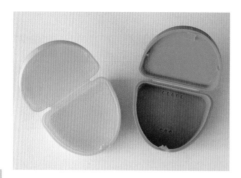

Figure 7.12 Appliance box.

- *Articulating forceps and articulating paper*
- *sharps box for excess trimmed wire*
- *hand mirror (if you need to demonstrate to the patient)*
- *appliance box (Figure 7.12), for use when the patient is playing sport, a musical instrument by mouth, etc.*
- *patient's model box as you need to put the work models in after treatment*
- *leaflet*

The nurse needs to:

- *supply personal protective equipment for the patient and staff*
- *make the patient comfortable*
- *have a straight handpiece and acrylic trimming bur ready*
- *have articulating paper and Miller's forceps ready*
- *have a hand mirror easily accessible*
- *reassure patient, when the brace is fitted, and let the patient see themselves*
- *encourage the patient to talk as it will feel strange and interfere with speech at first*
- *give the patient advice on eating*
- *give instructions on how to take the brace in and out and encourage the patient to try this themselves*
- *get the patient to do this so that the parents can see this being done*
- *discuss times it may need to be removed, supply protective case for these times*
- *discuss problems which might arise from the patient playing instruments by mouth, i.e. wind instruments*
- *give instructions on how to clean the appliance (it is helpful to advise the patient to fill the basin with water before they clean the appliance as it will 'bounce' on the surface of the water if dropped rather than fracture on impact with a porcelain basin)*
- *discuss the use of a mouth guard for contact sports*
- *give lots of positive feedback on how it looks (this can worry patients)*

REMOVABLE APPLIANCES

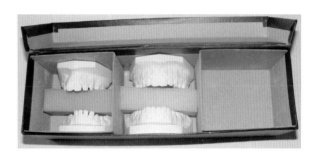

Figure 7.13 Pre- and posttreatment study models in box.

- *check that the patient understands what to do if they are actively turning screws, etc.*
- *give the patient the turning key in a secure bag*
- *go through the leaflet again (give them another one if it is lost)*
- *file the Medical Devices form for the appliance in the patient's notes*
- *make sure the patient has a number for advice (in an emergency)*

At subsequent appointments, you need the same tray set up.

You also need to check with the patient that there are no problems with the brace. If there are problems and the brace is not being worn as instructed, then there will be little progress.

Some patients have problems:

- with discomfort caused by the brace (sore areas of the mouth)
- with the idea of wearing it (they don't want to comply)
- with social difficulties (teasing from friends, difficulty speaking in school)

You can usually tell if a brace is not being worn enough if:

- *it looks shiny and new*
- *there are few indentations in the mouth, e.g. on palatal soft tissue*
- *there is difficulty taking it in and out (not a practiced skill)*
- *it affects speech (sounds like they are sucking a sweet)*

If this is the case, rather than ask a closed question:

- *'Have you been wearing your brace?'*

ask:

- *'What do you find difficult about wearing your brace?'*

or

- *'When can't you wear your brace?'*

At the completion of treatment, final impressions will need to be taken.
These are cast and trimmed as study models.

If there is to be no further treatment, these need to go, with the initial set of study models (Figure 7.13) to be PAR scored. (This PAR scoring is explained in Chapter 3 on Occlusal indices.)

Often, removable appliances are used prior to fixed appliance therapy. If so, the patient will need to wear the appliance in a passive mode until the 'train tracks' are fitted.

Chapter 8

Transpalatal arches, lingual arches and quad helix

The transpalatal arch, lingual arch and quad helix are fixed appliances that are:

- fitted on teeth, most commonly on molar teeth, using bands
- usually part of standard fixed appliance therapy

The transpalatal arch and lingual arch are used to maintain space.

Sometimes, when Ds and Es are lost and their permanent successors are slow to erupt, the first permanent molars drift forwards, into the space.

This can happen if there is early loss due to caries, etc., which would mean that the successor tooth was not ready to erupt and the space would need to be held for some time.

This space may also be used:

- To correct mild anterior crowding
- To reinforce anchorage by holding the banded molar teeth in position while active fixed appliance treatment progresses
- To allow consolidation of the developing occlusion

If there is to be a delay in starting the next phase, after preliminary molar movements and perhaps while awaiting eruption of teeth, a transpalatal arch can be fitted. This can be used as a holding device and can be retained right up until such time as heavy gauge wires in the fixed appliances can then maintain the molar positions.

The transpalatal or lingual arch consists of:

- molar bands cemented onto the first molars
- a fitted arch across the palate or lingually to the lower teeth and extending to the lower first molars
- the upper arch often has a pad of acrylic at its centre, known as a Nance button, which prevents it from pressing onto the palate

The bar can be either

- soldered to the bands in the laboratory

or

- fitted into a palatal or lingual tube on the band

MAKING AND FITTING OF ARCHES

For this treatment,
  at the first appointment, the nurse will need to prepare:

- *the patient's clinical notes*
- *mouth mirror*
- *dental floss*
- *posterior separating modules*
- *separating module pliers*

Procedure:

- *The nurse ensures that everyone is wearing personal protective equipment*
- *The patient is seated comfortably in the chair*
- *The patient is then told what is to happen and what the aim is, i.e. why this is happening and what it is going to achieve*
- Using separating module pliers, elastic rings are placed either side of the molar around which the bands are to be fitted (This is done several days in advance of fitting the bands as it 'springs' the teeth a tiny space apart which makes it easier for the clinician and more comfortable for the patient when trying on the bands)
- *The patient is then told what to expect over the next few days:*
  - *that it may be painful around the molar teeth for about 24–48 hours*
  - *what to do if a 'ring' falls out*
  - *that if it is swallowed, it will not be harmful*
  - *how to clean their teeth without dislodging the separating rings*

On the second visit, the nurse will need to prepare:

- *clinical notes*
- *study model box*
- *mirror, probe, College tweezers*
- *trays of appropriate molar bands*
- *bite stick*
- *floss*
- *Mershon pusher or plugger*
- *impression trays*
- *alginate, bowl, spatula (putty, if preferred)*
- *receiver for gagging reflex*
- *posterior separating modules*
- *separating module pliers*

- *laboratory instruction sheet*
- *plastic bag, label and disinfectant for impression*

Procedure:

- The nurse must *ensure that everyone is wearing personal protective equipment*
- *The patient is made comfortable in the chair*
- A probe is used to remove the separating modules one by one (it is important to make sure that all separators are taken out as, if accidentally left, they can cause periodontal problems. For this reason, many elastic separators are radiopaque)
- Floss is used between the teeth to remove any debris
- The correct size of band for each tooth is selected
- These are fitted and contoured to the teeth using a Mershon pusher/plugger and bite stick, and left on the teeth
- An alginate or putty impression is taken with the bands in position
- The impression is removed from the mouth
- The bands are then removed from the teeth and placed back in their correct position in the impression
- The separating modules are replaced between the teeth either side of the first molars to maintain the space
- *The impression is placed in disinfectant*
- *The laboratory instruction is written*
- *This then goes to the laboratory where the impression is cast*
- *The palatal or lingual bar is fabricated and the bands usually soldered to it*

For the third appointment to fit the palatal/lingual arch(es), *the nurse will need to prepare:*

- *the patient's clinical notes*
- *the patient's study models*
- *work models with arches soldered to bands*
- *mirror, probe and College tweezers*
- *dental floss*
- *handpiece and prophylactic paste*
- *cheek expander*
- *cement powder and liquid*
- *pad and spatula*
- *3-in-1 syringe*
- *aspirator tube*
- *cotton wool rolls*
- *bite stick*
- *Mershon pusher/plugger*
- *Mitchell trimmer*
- *sharps box*

Procedure:

- *The nurse ensures that everyone is wearing personal protective equipment*
- *The patient is made comfortable in the chair*
- The separators are removed
- Floss is used to clear any debris
- The bands and arch are tried in to check the fit is satisfactory
- The cheek expander is put in
- The teeth are cleaned using prophylactic paste, rubber cup and contra-angled handpiece
- The teeth are isolated and, with the palatal or lingual arch, are dried
- Cement is mixed and put into the inside of the molar bands
- The bands and palatal/lingual arch are put into position
- All traces of excess cement are removed
- *Check for patient comfort*
- *The patient is given instructions on oral hygiene*
- *Explanatory leaflet outlining dietary restrictions, etc. is given to the patient*
- *The Medical Devices form from the laboratory is filed in the patient's notes*

There needs to be the appropriate tray of instruments for these procedures available, when required.

Palatal and lingual arches are kept in position in the mouth until the clinician decides that they are no longer needed.

When they need to be removed, the molar bands are lifted off and then replaced without the palatal/lingual arch, if the treatment is to continue.

REMOVAL OF ARCHES

The nurse will need to prepare:

- *the patient's clinical notes*
- *the patient's model box*
- *mirror, probe and College tweezers*
- *posterior band removing pliers*
- *band slitting pliers*
- *Mitchell trimmer*
- *3-in-1 syringe*
- *handpiece, rubber cup and prophylactic paste*
- *aspirator tubes*
- *sharps box*

TRANSPALATAL ARCHES, LINGUAL ARCHES AND QUAD HELIX

Procedure:

- *The nurse needs to ensure that everyone is wearing personal protective equipment*
- *The patient is made comfortable in the chair*
- Using posterior band removing pliers, the band is gently eased off each tooth
- Band slitting pliers are used to cut the band if this is preferred
- Any cement residue is cleaned off using a Mitchell trimmer
- Using a handpiece, rubber cup and prophy paste, the teeth are cleaned
- *Discarded arch and bands are disposed of in the sharps box*

QUAD HELIX

A quad helix (Figure 8.1) has some similarities with palatal and lingual arches.

The main difference is that it is an active device, usually used to expand the width of the upper dental arch.

It derives its name from:

- quad, meaning four
- helix, meaning circle

Instead of having one heavy gauge wire loop in the palate, there is a continuous length of wire into which are bent four circles which make the wire very springy.

It is an appliance that is fixed to the teeth using molar bands.

In the laboratory, the device is attached to molar bands which have been selected and tried in by the clinician.

Following this, a work model is cast with the molar bands placed on it.

The quad helix wire is then fabricated by the technician and soldered to the molar bands on their palatal side. (Palatal tubes for a removable quad helix can alternatively be used.)

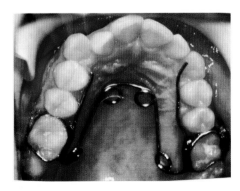

Figure 8.1 Quad helix cemented in place.

TRANSPALATAL ARCHES, LINGUAL ARCHES AND QUAD HELIX

This is then cemented by following the same process as for a palatal arch but is activated by expanding the quad helix beforehand.

The active spring then exerts pressure laterally and widens the arch transversely.

For the first *appointment, the nurse needs to prepare:*

- *the patient's clinical notes*
- *the patient's model box*
- *mirror, probe and College tweezers*
- *posterior separating modules*
- *separating module insertion pliers*
- *dental floss*

Procedure:

- *The nurse ensures that the dentist, nurse and patient wear personal protective equipment*
- *The patient is made comfortable in the chair*
- Separating modules are loaded on to the pliers
- *One is placed on each side (i.e. mesially and distally) of each molar tooth which is to have a band fitted onto it*
- *The patient is given an instruction leaflet*
- *The patient is advised on:*
  - *what to do when cleaning near the separating rings, i.e. brush, not floss*
  - *what to do if the ring comes out, as there is no need to panic*
  - *what foods to avoid, e.g. to avoid a very sticky or chewy diet*
  - *what to do if there is any discomfort – just to take a mild analgesic*

Some patients get very worried if they think that they have swallowed a separating ring. Reassure them that if they have done so, it will not do them any harm.

For the second appointment, the nurse needs to prepare:

- *the patient's clinical notes*
- *the patient's model box*
- CA *handpiece, rubber cup and prophy paste*
- *3-in-1 syringe*
- *aspirator tip*
- *trays of appropriate molar bands*
- *Mershon pusher/plugger*
- *bite stick*
- *upper impression tray*
- *alginate, bowl and spatula (putty, if preferred)*
- *bowl, in case of gagging reflex*
- *tissues and mouthwash*
- *solution to disinfect the impressions*
- *the laboratory instruction sheet*

Procedure:

- *The nurse needs to ensure that the dentist, nurse and patient are wearing personal, protective equipment*
- *The patient is seated comfortably*
- The separating rings are removed
- Floss is used to remove any debris
- The bands are selected and fitted and contoured by using Mershon pusher/plugger and/or bite stick
- The impression is taken with the bands in place
- The impression is removed and the bands placed in the correct position in the impression
- *The impression is disinfected, labelled and bagged*
- *The laboratory sheet is written and the impression sent to the technician*
- The separating modules are replaced

At the next visit, *the nurse needs to prepare:*

- *the patient's model box*
- *the patient's work from the laboratory*
- *cement, powder and liquid*
- *CA handpiece, prophylactic paste and rubber cup*
- *pad and spatula*
- *3-in-1 syringe*
- *aspirator*
- *cotton wool rolls*

Procedure:

- *Ensure that the patient, clinician and nurse are wearing personal protective equipment*
- *The patient is made comfortable in the chair*
- *The patient's models and appliance are ready*
- *The patients Medical Devices form is filed into the notes*
- The separating modules are removed and the areas flossed
- With handpiece, rubber cup and paste, the teeth are cleaned
- The quad helix is tried in to check that it is satisfactory and activated
- Teeth and quad helix are dried
- Cement is mixed and used to cover inside of bands, then the quad helix is seated
- The patient is made to bite on damp cotton wool rolls, applying pressure until cement begins to set
- any excess cement is removed
- Check the patient is comfortable
- *The patient is given instruction on diet, oral hygiene, etc.*
- *The patient is given the information leaflet*

TRANSPALATAL ARCHES, LINGUAL ARCHES AND QUAD HELIX

The quad helix may need a number of adjustments to achieve the upper arch expansion before this stage is completed.

REMOVAL OF THE QUAD HELIX

This is a procedure which is similar to that used when taking out transpalatal or lingual arches.

- Using posterior band removing pliers or band slitters, the bands are eased off the teeth
- The residual cement is cleaned off
- The molar bands are replaced by either
  - re-cementing new bands
    or
  - cutting the quad helix off the original bands and re-cementing those

NB: If used bands are re-cemented, the bands must be smoothed and polished to make sure that they are not rough to the tongue.

Quad helix expansion is a preliminary phase prior to full fixed appliance therapy.

Chapter 9
Rapid maxillary expansion

When the maxilla and the mandible do not 'match' together, it can cause a transverse malocclusion.

This occlusal problem is a discrepancy between:

- a narrow or V-shaped upper dental arch form and a U-shaped lower arch

In this case, it means that the upper buccal segment teeth are in bilateral crossbite.

In order to correct the bite, the upper jaw needs to be expanded (Figure 9.1). Rapid maxillary expansion (RME) (Figure 9.2) devices are:

- fixed – cemented onto the buccal segment teeth which incorporates a central expansion screw

The appliance:

- It works by rapidly expanding the palate, the bone of which is divided in two halves by a midline suture
- The appliance is cemented to teeth on each side
- These are joined together by an expansion screw
- The space between the two halves is initially small
- Each time the screw is turned, this space gets wider
- This can be done on patients in late mixed or second dentition up to about 15 years of age

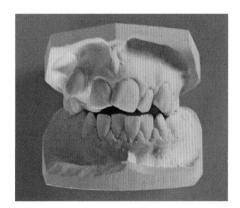

Figure 9.1 Models of case before fitting rapid maxillary expansion.

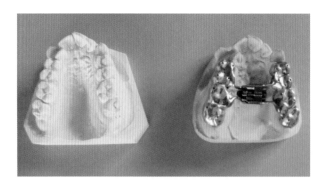

Figure 9.2 Silver casting
rapid maxillary expansion
appliance with model.

This has similarities to distraction osteogenesis (where the bone is surgically cut prior to expansion). The gap between the two sections of bone (in the case of the palate, the midline) must fill in and consolidate with new bone.

By turning the midline palatal screw a quarter circle turn twice daily, the upper arch widens. Patients often feel slight discomfort in the palate.

Depending on the manufacturers instructions, the number of quarter circle turns might be 40, comprising two quarter circle turns per day for 20 days.

This is followed by a passive period of 2–3 months to allow consolidation of the bone in the palate. During this time the device is left in the mouth.

When it is removed, impressions are taken and a Hawley retainer made to maintain the position achieved. This must be fitted as soon as possible to prevent relapse of the expansion.

RME devices can be made of:

- acrylic
- silver (Figure 9.3)
- soldered to bands on first permanent molars and usually pre-molars

and are made in the dental laboratory.

Unlike removable expansion appliances, they cannot be removed by the patient.

The first appointment would be for **impressions**.

The nurse needs to prepare:

- *the patient's clinical notes*
- *upper and lower impression trays*
- *alginate, bowl and spatula*
- *wax or material for bite registration*
- *wax knife*
- *method of softening wax, blow torch, flame, hot water*
- *bowl for gagging reflex*

RAPID MAXILLARY EXPANSION

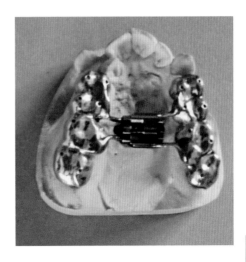

Figure 9.3 Silver casting rapid maxilliary expansion appliance close-up.

- *tissues and mouthwash*
- *solution to disinfect impressions and bite*
- *laboratory worksheets*
- *plastic bags*
- *camera (if necessary, then also lip retractors)*

and to assist the clinician at the chairside procedure, the nurse needs to:

- *ensure that the patient and staff are wearing personal protective equipment*
- *seat the patient comfortably in the chair*
- *choose the impression tray sizes carefully*
- *use beading wax to extend the tray if necessary*
- *record wax bite*
- *mix lower then upper alginate impressions (putty impressions, if preferred)*
- *provide the patient with mouthwash and tissues*
- *soak impressions in disinfectant tank*
- *put the impressions and bite into plastic bag with the name of the patient*
- *prepare instruction sheet with instructions to go with the impressions to the laboratory*
- *check whether the patient and technician have details of the date and time of next appointment*

Before the appliance is fitted, the patient and the person who will be turning the screw for them must have clear instructions and a demonstration of how the screw on the appliance works. This is done as a 'dry run' on the appliance before cementing it into the mouth. Several practice runs must be made to make sure this is understood and works correctly.

FITTING THE APPLIANCE

The nurse needs to prepare:

- *the patient's notes*
- *the model box*
- *appliance*
- *key to turn the expansion screw*
- *mouth mirror*
- *probe*
- *College tweezers*
- *cement, pad and spatula*
- *Mitchell trimmer*
- *camera (if photographs are required)*
- *cheek/lip retractors*
- *photographic mirrors*
- *3-in-1 tips*
- *cotton wool rolls*
- *aspirator/saliva ejector*
- *plastic bag or box for key*
- *hand mirror*
- *leaflet*

and to assist the clinician at the chairside procedure:

- ensure that the patient and staff are wearing appropriate protection
- ensure that the patient is sitting comfortably
- allow the appliance to be tried in and the method of turning the screw explained and demonstrated until everyone is fully confident
- keep the teeth dry
- prepare 3-in-1 suction, cotton wool rolls
- *dry the fitting surfaces of the appliance*
- *mix the cement and fill all the fitting surfaces of the appliance*
- *on cementing, supply two damp cotton rolls for the patient to bite on*
- *clear off excess cement gingivally with Mitchell trimmer*
- *provide the patient with mouthwash and tissues*
- *show the patient the appliance in the mouth in the hand mirror*
- *take intra-oral and extra-oral photographs (if required)*
- *reassure the patient that although it feels strange they will soon get used to it and give them cleaning and dietary advice*
- *advise them that there is going to be a large gap opening up between the central incisors as the expansion progresses*
- *give a leaflet to the patient and their accompanying person*

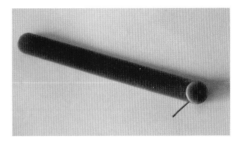

Figure 9.4 Safety swivel key.

- *give them the key (Figure 9.4) used to turn the screw (ask the accompanying person to check that they can see the screw hole and fit the key into it while the patient lies flat as this is how they will need to do it at home)*
- *file the Medical Devices form in the patient's notes*
- *ask the patient to keep a diary of their progress with screw adjustments*
- *check that there is an appointment arranged in 3 weeks time*

THE NEXT APPOINTMENT – WHEN THE SCREW TURNING HAS BEEN COMPLETED

The nurse needs to prepare:

- *mirror*
- *probe*
- *College tweezers*
- *ruler*
- *dividers*

and to assist the clinician at the chairside procedure:

- *ensure that dentist, patient and nurse are wearing personal protective equipment*
- *make sure that the patient is sitting comfortably*
- check that the correct number of turns has been completed and that the screw has not been adjusted beyond that number
- make sure that the device is still secure, that expansion has occurred
- make sure that a marked upper diastema (centre line space between the front teeth; Figure 9.5) has appeared

Some clinicians like to take more photographs at this point.

A further appointment is made for 2–3 months ahead to remove the RME and make and fit a retainer.

RAPID MAXILLARY EXPANSION

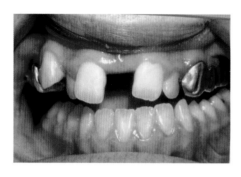

Figure 9.5 Diastema after rapid maxilliary expansion appliance treatment.

When the palate has consolidated, *the nurse needs to prepare:*

- *the patient's notes*
- *the patient's model box*
- *laboratory sheets*
- *mirror*
- *probe*
- *Mitchell trimmer*
- *hand mirror*
- *posterior band removing pliers*
- *alginate, bowl and spatula*
- *impression trays*
- *wax or registration material*
- *method of softening wax, blow torch, flame or hot water*
- *impression disinfection solution*
- *bowl in case of gagging reflex*
- *plastic bag*

and to assist the clinician at the chairside procedure:

- *ensure that the patient and staff are wearing appropriate protection*
- *make sure that the patient is seated comfortably*
- remove the RME and discard in appropriate waste (*if the RME is made of silver, disinfect and return to the laboratory*)
- remove any residual cement from the teeth
- take upper and lower alginate impressions
- record bite
- *disinfect and bag impressions*

Instructions are given to the technician to make study models, needed to record the end of this stage of treatment, and a passive Hawley retainer, to maintain the expansion achieved. (It is essential that this retainer is fitted the same, or the next day, otherwise, the maxillary arch expansion will begin to relapse very quickly.)

RAPID MAXILLARY EXPANSION

FITTING THE RETAINER

The nurse will need to prepare:

- *clinical notes*
- *the patient's model box*
- *mirror, probe and College tweezers*
- *Hawley retainer appliance*
- *Adams pliers*
- *instruction leaflet*
- *straight handpiece*
- *acrylic burs*
- *retainer case*

and to assist the clinician at the chairside procedure:

- *ensure that dentist, patient and nurse are wearing personal protective equipment*
- *make sure the patient is sitting comfortably*

The orthodontist will make sure:

- the appliance fits comfortably and is secure (adjust if necessary)
- the patient is shown how to take it in and out of the mouth (using hand mirror)

The nurse will:

- *give instructions on how to clean it (back up by giving a leaflet)*
- *advise that it is to be worn day and night, removed only for cleaning*
- *supply a retainer case*
- *name and date work and study models and put into the model box*
- *file the Medical Devices form for appliance in the patient's notes*

The timing of the next appointment will depend on whether it is to check the retainer or to proceed direct to the next stage of treatment.

RAPID MAXILLARY EXPANSION

Chapter 10

Extra-oral traction and extra-oral anchorage

Of all the appliances, this is the one most patients like least.

Extra-oral traction (EOT) is also known as headgear. It uses positive directional force and the anchorage is from the back of the head or neck.

To get the patient to wear it as instructed for the correct amount of time means that they need to be well motivated and compliant.

It is the only appliance that is worn which has a very visible component because it is worn outside the mouth.

As it is so visible, many patients are willing to wear it while they are at home but are reluctant to wear it to school or on social occasions.

The design of the head cap has now been greatly improved and efforts have been made to make it more patient-friendly. They now come in a range of bright colours and denim material, but this has not changed the general attitude (Figure 10.1).

It can be worn in conjunction with both:

- removable appliances
- fixed appliances

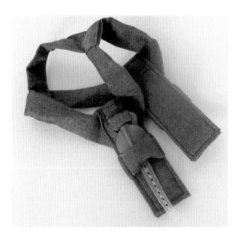

Figure 10.1 Head cap.

The time scale for wear varies and may be:

- full-time
- 14 hours a day
- just overnight, when asleep for extra oral anchorage (EOA)

It can be used:

- to reinforce anchorage (to prevent the upper molars coming forward)
- to retract the upper buccal segments (to make enough room anteriorly)

If teeth may need to be extracted, it would normally be at the back of the dental arch to facilitate distal movement.

Apart from what is normally thought of as headgear, there is a system called reverse-pull headgear. This system aims to advance the maxillary teeth rather than move them backwards and is used in Class lll cases. It requires the use of a face frame for anchorage.

However, it is not used as much as headgear, which aims to distalise or to retain the upper buccal segments to stop them coming forward.

Head caps can have a backward and upward pull.

Cervical (neck) straps rest on the back of the neck and have not only a backward but also a downward pull.

What it looks like

For conventional EOT, there are several different types of head cap and cervical strap available, made from plastic or fabric, with a metal bow.

The face bow

A strong wire component that connects the intra-oral appliance to the extra-oral device.

How the headgear is assembled

- The upper appliance (if removable) is fitted in the mouth
- The inner bow of the face bow is inserted into the buccal tubes soldered to the first permanent molar cribs on the appliance in the mouth
- The preformed head cap is fitted over the head
- Attached at the side of the cap in front of the ears are attachments for two sprung C modules which fit onto the sides of the head cap
- These modules are assembled
- The straps which are attached to them have a series of holes

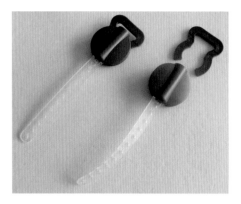

Figure 10.2 C modules.

- The outer bow of the face bow is lateral to the cheeks and terminates in hooks to which are fitted the C module straps
- The same level of hole must be used on each side of the head to maintain equal forces
- The headgear and face bow are checked for patient comfort and correct position

In recent years, there has been great concern regarding safety when wearing these devices. These now have safety features that make them less likely to become dislodged and cause an injury to the face, and more particularly the eyes.

Clinicians strongly advise that a Masel strap should always be worn, particularly when the patient is involved in close contact with other people. This is attached on one external hook and passed around the back of the neck and attached on the other one. This makes it harder to dislodge. 'C' modules also have safety features as they spring apart if suddenly pulled too hard (if it were to be done accidentally) (Figure 10.2).

The face bows have features on the inner bow which help prevent the bow being accidentally pulled from buccal tubes.

FITTING HEADGEAR

When the patient is having headgear fitted, *the nurse needs to prepare:*

- *the patient's clinical notes*
- *the patient's model box*
- *if a removable appliance is being used, ensure it is ready in the surgery*
- *mouth mirror*

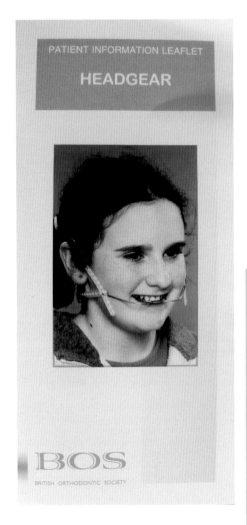

Figure 10.3 BOS leaflet. (Reproduced with the kind permission of the British Orthodontic Society.)

- *Mauns heavy-duty cutters*
- *Adams pliers*
- *spring-forming pliers*
- *ruler*
- *face bow (Figure 10.4) with safety locking device*
- *the C modules (these contain coil springs for force application)*
- *disposable wire markers*
- *sharps box for excess cut off wire*
- *a hand mirror*
- patient information leaflet (Figure 10.3)

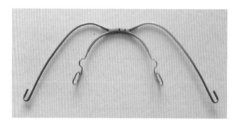

Figure 10.4 Face bow.

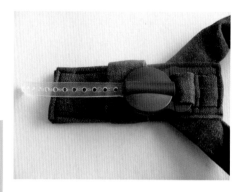

Figure 10.5 C modules fitted to head cap.

Fitting the ready-made cap

- *The patient is asked to choose the colour they would like*
- The correct size of face bow is selected (this should be a safety one for choice)
- A pair of Adams pliers is used to adjust this wire

Check that the bow fits well into the upper first molar tubes either of the fixed or the removable appliance. If the outer bow needs to be shortened, use Mauns heavy-duty cutters. Disposable wire markers can be used to mark the wire where it has to be cut and adjusted.

Ensure that the C modules (Figure 10.5) have a sufficient amount of pull. They have coil springs inside the module which apply continuous force.

Check that when these are tugged, e.g. if done accidentally, they would spontaneously release.

CHAIRSIDE FITTING PROCEDURE

With the chosen head cap to hand, the nurse should assist the clinician:

- *ensure that the patient and staff wear personal protection*
- *make sure that the patient is seated comfortably in the dental chair*

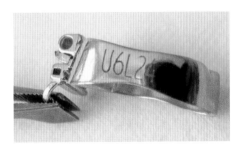

Figure 10.6 Band with tube for EOT.

- if being fitted to a fixed appliance, a face bow is fitted into the upper first molar (EOT) buccal tubes
- the bow must be adjusted so that it is well clear of the upper front teeth and does not interfere with the components of the fixed appliance near the buccal tubes
- *show the patient how to put on the head cap*
- *demonstrate how the head cap is connected to the outer bow via the 'C' modules on the head cap*
- *fit a Masel safety strap which fits over one end of the outer bow, round the back of the neck and over the other end. This is an extra precaution. Show the patient how this is taken on and off and when it should be used*
- *let the patient practice fitting the head cap and strapping themselves in several times until they feel confident*

When used with fixed appliances, the EOT tubes are alongside the fixed appliance arch wire tubes, as part of the welded attachment to the upper first molar bands (Figure 10.6). If the head cap is being fitted in conjunction with a removable appliance, the clinician will ensure that it fits comfortably and that the cribs have been adjusted for adequate retention.

When the appliance is out of the patient's mouth, show the patient how to fit the ends of the inner bow into the tubes soldered to the upper first molar cribs.

The patient can then put the combined bow and removable appliance into their mouth.

Then, show the patient how to attach the head cap.

For safety reasons, with all headgear always impress on the patient,

Never put the head cap on or off with the bow attached.

Never take a removable appliance out until the cap has been removed.

The patient must practice and be able to assemble and remove the headgear.

The patient or the clinician must hold and stabilise the face bow with one hand whilst connecting or disconnecting the traction system with the other.

Full instructions must be given, reinforced by a written leaflet detailing:

- *how to look after the head cap*
- *for how long it must be worn each day*

- *when it should not be worn, e.g. hair washing*
- *how it is to be kept clean*

Patients are often encouraged to fill in headgear charts or to keep a diary to record the number of hours per day that the headgear is worn.

Wearing EOA as part of appliance therapy is usually to prevent the upper first molars from coming forward. Because there is no need to distalise the teeth, merely to keep them in their normal position, the hours of night time wear alone is sufficient.

For patients where there is a need to pull the upper buccal teeth distally, in order to gain space for the anterior teeth, there must be more hours of EOT per day.

Patients who wear it in conjunction with fixed and removable appliances have routine appointments and the headgear is adjusted at the same time.

Patients who wear extra-oral systems are requested to bring these at their routine adjustment appointments during treatment together with their diary of the number of hours of wear achieved each day.

Patients must be given a lot of encouragement.

There can never be too much praise.

If possible, there should be a guideline given to the patient as to how long this appliance may be needed, but a lot depends on their cooperation.

The nurse needs to prepare for all subsequent appointments for extra-oral adjustments:

- *the patient's clinical notes*
- *the patient's model box*
- *mouth mirror*
- *spring-forming pliers*
- *Adams pliers*
- *ruler*
- *Mauns heavy wire cutters*
- *disposable arch wire markers*
- *hand mirror*
- *sharps box*

EXTRA-ORAL TRACTION AND
EXTRA-ORAL ANCHORAGE

Chapter 11

Functional appliances

THE PROBLEM

These appliances are mainly used when correction is needed in Class II mal-occlusions. Their aim is to encourage forward development of the mandible which can reduce a significantly increased overjet (horizontal distance between the upper and lower incisor teeth) and correct a Class II molar relation to Class I.

When a patient comes into the surgery concerned that their upper teeth appear to 'stick out', they may also have:

- an underdeveloped mandible (and also a receding chin)
- a lower lip that curls under the upper teeth, often becoming trapped behind them

This makes the upper incisors seem to protrude even further.

A clinical assessment often shows that the front teeth are not positioned too far forward in relation to the upper face.

The problem is that the lower jaw has not grown sufficiently and is shorter than the upper.

The clinician may therefore decide that functional appliance therapy is needed.

They are designed to harness the power of the jaw and facial muscles to correct the occlusal relationship between the upper and lower arches. They hold the 'postured' mandible forward and are most effective in a growing patient.

They can therefore be used in the later mixed dentition through puberty to about 14 years of age.

In very severe cases of jaw-length discrepancy, particularly in older patients, orthognathic treatment (an osteotomy) is a treatment option.

For less severe cases and when the patient is still growing, functional appliance therapy is often the treatment of choice.

Most functional appliances (Figure 11.1) are removable and can be taken in and out for eating and cleaning.

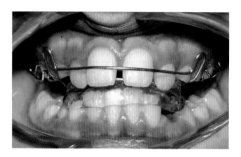

Figure 11.1 Functional appliance.

However, the success of these appliances is related to the compliance of the patient in wearing them as advised.

Patients who wear them intermittently make slow progress and, if treatment is not completed, can find that this can quickly relapse.

THE SOLUTION

The functional appliance works by movement of the teeth and alveolar bone with some forward mandibular development too.

They rely on oro-facial muscles to supply the force which, transmitted through the functional appliance, produces intermaxillary traction.

Before the appliance is fitted, the overjet is measured and recorded and this is done again at the end of treatment.

When the treatment is completed, it should be possible to gradually remove the appliance and find that the mandible and occlusion remain stable.

TYPES OF FUNCTIONAL APPLIANCE

There are many types of functional appliance. Because there seems to be no accepted classification of functional appliances many are known by the name of the clinician who developed them.

For example

the **Andresen** activator:

- is a tooth-borne appliance
- is basically an upper and lower appliance fused together, where the lower one is advanced forward of the upper
- is made of acrylic and wire
- is successful on Class II/I cases with well-aligned arches

FUNCTIONAL APPLIANCES

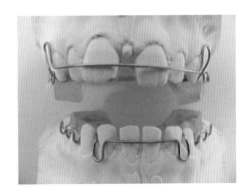

Figure 11.2 Clark Twin Block front view.

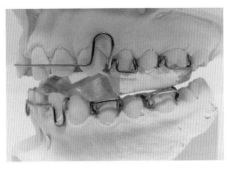

Figure 11.3 Clark Twin Block side view.

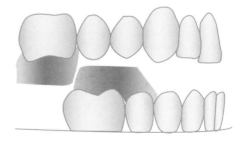

Figure 11.4 Diagram of position of blocks.

the **Frankel** function regulator:

- is a soft-tissue-borne appliance
- has lip and cheek bumpers
- is made of acrylic and wire
- is used in mixed and early second dentition

the **Clark Twin Block** (Figures 11.2–11.5):

- is a tooth-borne appliance
- is made of acrylic and wire
- is in two separate parts
- is worn on the upper and lower arches
- has close fitting base plates which makes it well tolerated

FUNCTIONAL APPLIANCES

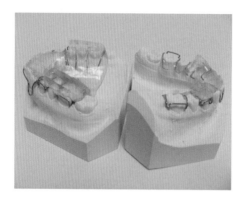

Figure 11.5 View of appliance on upper and lower model.

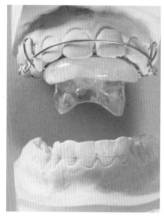

Figure 11.6 MOA showing rest for lower teeth in the postured position.

- has angled bite blocks which posture the mandible forward and the two parts slide over one another
- night-time wear of extra-oral traction (headgear) can be worn with this appliance
- is very popular with patients in the UK

the **Harvold** appliance:

- is a tooth-borne appliance
- is made of acrylic and wire
- holds the bite well open

the **Medium Open Activator** (MOA) (Figure 11.6):

- is a tooth-borne appliance
- is made of acrylic and wire comprising:
  - upper base plate
  - labial bow
  - cribs for retention

FUNCTIONAL APPLIANCES

- lower acrylic extension into which the lower incisors bite to posture the mandible
- has a smaller mandibular component
- is easier to wear

These functional appliances are all **removable** appliances

The Herbst functional appliance is an appliance which is **fixed** to the teeth
The Herbst appliance:

- is sometimes used when there is poor compliance and the patient will not wear a removable appliance for sufficient hours to make it effective
- is made with upper and lower components which are connected by telescopic pistons
- because of the easy range of vertical and some lateral movement, the appliance is well tolerated and comfortable to wear
- being cemented in place means that the patient has no option but to wear it full time, ensuring a higher level of success

These appliances call for a high degree of compliance in a well-motivated patient. The choice of functional appliance used depends on factors in the malocclusion and the personal preference of the orthodontist.

What the nurse needs to prepare for the first appointment

- *clinical notes*
- *Orthopantogram/lateral cephalometric radiographs*
- *mouth mirror*
- *alginate, bowls and spatula (putty (vinyl polysiloxane) if preferred)*
- *upper and lower impression trays*
- *wax (and occlusal registration bite recorders if required)*
- *method of softening wax, blow torch, hot water, etc.*
- *supply of cold water in container to chill the wax bite*
- *mouthwash and tissues*
- *solution to disinfect impressions and bite*
- *plastic bag and gauze*
- *laboratory instruction card*
- *clinical camera*
- *lip and cheek retractors*
- *photographic mirrors*
- *next date for fitting appointment*
- *information leaflet about functional appliances for patient (Figure 11.7)*

FUNCTIONAL APPLIANCES

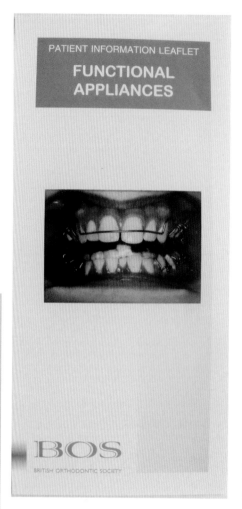

Figure 11.7 BOS leaflet. (Reproduced with the kind permission of the British Orthodontic Society.)

Procedure

The nurse:

- *ensures that everyone is wearing personal protective equipment*
- *makes sure the patient is comfortable*
- takes intra-oral and extra-oral photographs
- takes bite in normal centric occlusion (as the patient bites)
- takes another bite in the postured position using several thicknesses of wax (with the mandible biting in a forward position)
- *has supply of cold water in a suitable container to hand (the bite must be removed from the mouth and cooled before trying it in again to check that there has been no distortion)*
- takes upper and lower alginate or putty impressions

- *disinfects impressions and bite before they go off to the laboratory*
- *takes written laboratory design instructions and diagram, along with sterilised impressions and bite to the technician*
- *gives the patient an information leaflet about the functional appliance*

At the fitting appointment

The nurse will need:

- *appliance to be fitted*
- *hand mirror*
- *patient's model box*
- *mouth mirror*
- *ruler*
- *Adams pliers*
- *straight handpiece and acrylic bur*
- *instruction leaflet*
- *functional appliance case*
- *hand mirror*

Chairside procedure

The nurse will then:

- *ensure that the dentist, nurse and patient wear personal protective equipment*
- *make the patient comfortable in the chair*
- *assist the clinician in fitting the appliance ensuring that it is firm and lower teeth fit comfortably into the appliance in the forward position*
- *show the patient how to remove and insert appliance correctly*
- *record the starting overjet with the appliance out of the mouth*
- *go over the information and instruction leaflets again*
- *give the patient a functional appliance case in which to keep the appliance when it is out of the mouth, e.g. cleaning, contact sports*
- *advise the patient and parent of the amount of overjet reduction being aimed for at the conclusion of this phase of treatment*
- *explain to patient how and when it is to be worn*
- *tell patient how to clean the brace (after every meal and weekly with special cleaner, e.g. Brace Mate)*
- *confirm arrangements for wearing brace if the patient plays instruments by mouth*
- *confirm arrangements if patient plays contact sports and wears a mouth guard*
- *advise the patient to keep a diary of times of wear*
- *ask the patient and the parent if they have any questions*

FUNCTIONAL APPLIANCES

At subsequent appointments:

- the same format is followed until the measurement of the overjet has reduced to that planned for
- the molar relation should also be checked that this is being corrected
- when the required measurement has been reached further impressions will be taken to record the end of that stage of treatment
- if the patient is then to have fixed appliance therapy, the functional appliance will be worn at nights only to hold the correction achieved until the fixed appliance is fitted.

Functional appliances cannot align irregular teeth or arches, so most patients then move into fixed appliance therapy.

Chapter 12
Temporary anchorage devices

WHAT THEY ARE

Orthodontic treatment and treatment philosophies are always moving forward. A relatively recent technique, the use of a temporary anchorage screw, has expanded the scope of clinical work and clinicians can now create an anchorage site where they need it.

Temporary anchorage devices (TADs) are also known as:

- mini screws
- mini implants

The TAD is made of a medical-grade titanium alloy. It is literally a screw that is inserted through the gum and into the alveolar bone.

WHAT THEY DO

In orthodontic treatment, some teeth are used for anchorage, from which a force is applied to the teeth to be moved. This may be in the same dental arch or the opposing one. However, they may not always be in the right position or at the right angle to do this. But, by fitting a small screw a more precise anchorage site can be chosen.

There is now an increased range of treatment available to the clinician when using fixed and immovable anchor points; these can be for diverse uses, such as correcting open bites, uprighting molars or closing spaces. Because the clinician can usually position the device where it is needed, it will optimise the results and increase the range of tooth movements achievable.

Extra anchorage points are also useful when:

- the existing teeth are not suitable or insufficient
- the force might not move the teeth correctly
- the teeth required are not present (hypodontia)

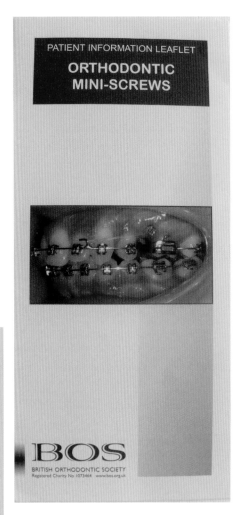

Figure 12.1 BOS leaflet on mini screws. (Reproduced with the kind permission of the British Orthodontic Society.)

The use of these devices also has advantages for patients. TADs are all intra-oral and the effectiveness of their treatment is improved.

THE ADVANTAGES OF TADs

The advantages of mini screws (Figure 12.1) are:

- they are quick and easy to use
- they have a success rate of over 75%
- they can be sited where the orthodontist thinks it will be of most benefit
- they can also provide an alternative to wearing headgear

- once fitted, they can be used straight away (no consolidation period)
- it is a relatively painless procedure, needing only a local anaesthetic on insertion
- they are screwed directly into the bone
- any mild discomfort lasts only a few days
- screws can safely be left in situ for several months
- screws are easily and painlessly removed
- once removed, the site heals quickly
- mini screws are relatively inexpensive

THE DISADVANTAGES OF TADs

The disadvantages of TADs are:

- they can fail
- they can become loose
- they can break
- on insertion, they can come into contact with a root
- the site can become infected
- the start-up cost of equipment

The added oral hygiene requirements for mini screws are basically:

- a chlorhexidine rinse for a week after insertion
- gentle manual brushing with fluoride toothpaste after meals while in place

It is possible to buy a kit which supplies the contra-angled hand driver, tips, screwdriver handle, screwdriver tips and a pilot drill. All attachments can be bought individually, including post heads, bracket head, contra-angled tips and screwdriver tips.

All screws come pre packed in sterilised or sterilisable envelopes.

Separate sterilisation trays are also sold with these kits.

HOW THE DEVICE IS FITTED

When the TAD is fitted (Figure 12.2) the patient will feel some discomfort, like a pressing feeling.

This passes off very quickly, but some clinicians like to apply a little topical anaesthetic to the area followed by a small local anaesthetic injection.

It takes only a few minutes to insert these devices (Figures 12.3 and 12.4), during which time the patient does not feel pain.

TEMPORARY ANCHORAGE DEVICES

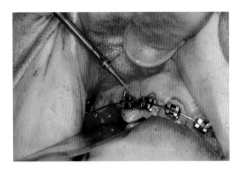

Figure 12.2 TAD being inserted. (Reproduced with the kind permission of Steve Jones, Eastman Dental Hospital, London.)

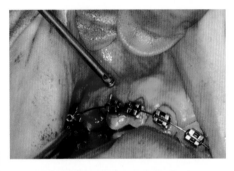

Figure 12.3 TAD fully inserted. (Reproduced with the kind permission of Steve Jones, Eastman Dental Hospital, London.)

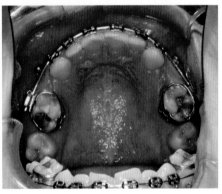

Figure 12.4 TAD in situ. (Reproduced with the kind permission of Steve Jones, Eastman Dental Hospital, London.)

However, it can be painful afterwards. This is not often severe and the patient is advised to take the same level of analgesic that they would if they had a headache.

The patient is given patient comfort wax or medical-grade silicone to use if the screw should cause irritation by rubbing the soft issues on the inside of the mouth.

Because the device is basically a screw, it is inserted using a screwdriver. When the time comes to remove the device, after putting a little topical anaesthetic on the gum around the site, the screwdriver turns the screw in the other direction and gently eases it out. This procedure takes roughly the same length of time as it does to put it in.

The advantages outweigh the disadvantages.

This is a technique that expands the scope of orthodontic treatment in a unique way.

It is a temporary measure, not intended to be used for long periods.

It is user-friendly, easy-to-fit and ready-to-use straight away.

The procedure must take place using sterile techniques.

The screw is made of titanium alloy and has different lengths and thicknesses depending in which part of the mouth it is to be inserted.

- The longest (10 mm) screw is for areas of thick bone:
  - the infra-zygomatic crest
  - the molar regions of the mandible
- The middle size (8 mm) screw is for facial and palatal areas of the maxilla:
  - tooth-bearing areas of the mandible
- The smallest size (6 mm) screw is for the facial area of the maxilla:
  - tooth-bearing areas of the mandible

The clinician selects which one is most appropriate to use and decides what is to be attached to the device, e.g.:

- thread elastic
- linked chain
- coil
- NiTi coil spring

What the nurse needs to prepare for fitting a TAD:

- the patient's clinical notes
- the patient's radiographs and models
- mirror, probe and College tweezers
- a small pledget of cotton wool
- gel for topical anaesthesia (and cartridge syringe, disposable needle and ampoule, if local injection is to be given)
- tray set-up for the procedure taking place
- 3-in-1 syringe
- aspirator
- lip expander
- cotton wool rolls
- a fixed appliance tray and sundries to adjust the appliance
- a TAD fitting tray
- tissues and a glass of mouthwash
- sharps box
- hand mirror
- instruction leaflet on oral hygiene
- box of relief wax or medical-grade relief silicone

TEMPORARY ANCHORAGE DEVICES

For the procedure, the nurse needs to assist the clinician at the chairside:

- *ensure that the patient and staff all wear personal protection*
- *seat the patient comfortably in the chair*
- *ensure that access to the site is clear*
- *make sure that the anchorage-fitting kit is laid out ready*
- *make sure that the method of attaching the screw to the fixed appliance is ready to use, e.g. coil, springs or linked chain*
- *assist with a fixed appliance adjustment in addition to fitting the temporary screw*
- *give the patient an instruction leaflet on care of the device*
- *give the patient oral hygiene instructions*
- *make sure that the patient understands what the signs might be if something was not right and has the emergency telephone number*
- *make sure that the patient has the correct mouthwash and patient comfort wax*
- *give the patient the next appointment*

When these appliances have outlived their usefulness, they can be very easily removed. This:

- does not necessarily require an anaesthetic
- does not cause the patient pain
- the site heals very quickly
- leaves no lasting damage to bone or soft tissue

The use of these devices will expand many treatment options in the future. This may have particular implications in areas where specific and additional anchorage is needed, such as hypodontia cases.

Chapter 13

Fixed appliances – what they do and what is used

This chapter will concentrate on what is meant by fixed appliance therapy and what the nurse needs to prepare when either fitting or adjusting a fixed appliance in the surgery.

Fixed appliance therapy:

- moves teeth with great accuracy and control
- normally moves a number of teeth at the same time
- is more sophisticated than a removable appliance
- can move crowns and the roots of teeth bodily, not just tip them
- can be used with extraction or non-extraction treatments
- is sometimes used following removable or functional appliance treatment
- extra-oral traction (EOT) can be worn with it (e.g. night time to prevent first molars drifting forward)
- is used in conjunction with multi-disciplinary treatments such as orthognathic surgery and hypodontia cases
- cannot be taken in and out by the patient

PATIENT EXPECTATION – THE POPULAR CULTURE OF TRAIN TRACKS

When patients speak of orthodontic treatment, the majority of them think of fixed appliances (Figure 13.1), a system that they often refer to as 'train tracks'. A look at clinic lists would reveal a high proportion of 'fixed' adjustment appointments on them.

For most patients of normal orthodontic age, this is the appliance that they would all prefer if they had the choice.

It is regarded:

- as the gold standard, 'the proper brace'
- that braces that are removable are often seen by the patients as inferior
- as fashionable, most of their friends have it, and it gives them status

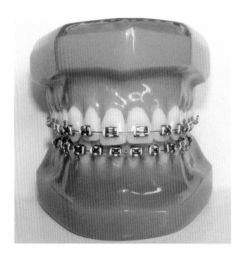

Figure 13.1 Upper and lower fixed appliances with metal brackets.

PEER PRESSURE

Much discussion of their treatment goes on at school break times and experiences are exchanged.

Most teenage patients like to be seen:

- as having the same appliances as their friends
- to be part of the crowd

However, for the patients who try to be seen as different, train tracks are also requested as they have 'alternative' role models, such as:

- Ugly Betty, the girl who does not fit in with the popular stereotype of a teenager

or

- Sid, the evil kid next door, the opposite of the stereotypical good guy, Andy, in Toy Story.

Patients have their own language when talking about fixed appliance treatment.
Apart from the system being known as 'train tracks', they call:

- the appliance – 'braces'
- the bands – 'rings'
- the brackets – 'blocks'

By definition, it is a system that is fixed to the teeth and one which the patient is not able to remove.

STAGES OF TREATMENT IN FIXED APPLIANCE THERAPY

There are four stages in fixed appliance therapy:

- Alignment – aligning irregular teeth including rotations, height differentials, etc.
- Working – resolving abnormal overbites and overjets and space closure after extractions
- Finishing– torquing incisors and fine aesthetic detailing
- Retention – maintenance of the treatment results with retainers

Fixed appliances can be fitted to the teeth either by:

- direct bonding
- indirect bonding

WHAT IS USED IN FIXED APPLIANCE THERAPY

The basic mechanics of 'train tracks' are:

- each tooth has an attachment fitted to it
- initially, a fine arch wire is fitted into these attachments
- the teeth can be moved along the wire into alignment or be moved by the flexibility of the arch wire itself

In order to do this, the system uses:

- bands (on molar teeth)
- brackets
- and/or buccal tubes (on molar teeth)

Brackets and buccal tubes are bonded to the teeth with composite adhesive and glass ionomer cements.

Molar bands are first fitted to the teeth and then cemented.

These provide 'handles' on the teeth which engage the arch wire.

The capability of fixed appliances is such that a finished result should include:

- a balanced occlusion (all teeth biting evenly together)
- no residual spacing
- no rotated or submerged teeth
- an acceptable gum line (the margins look even)

While removable appliances can expand arches and tip teeth, the fixed appliance is more sophisticated.

FIXED APPLIANCES – WHAT THEY DO AND WHAT IS USED

It has a great many applications and can achieve many kinds of tooth movement:

- positional
- rotational
- ability to extrude and intrude teeth
- ability to torque the roots

THE ATTACHMENTS

- bands
- brackets
- buccal tubes, buttons, eyelets and cleats

Bands

Bands are fitted exactly around a tooth, usually on the molars and being in the masticatory regions of the dentition provide extra strength. (In some cases, however, buccal tubes may be sufficient.)

They are (Figure 13.2):

- usually made of stainless steel
- pre-formed and come in a large range of sizes
- used on both first and second molars
- stored in separate trays, for each molar and for each quadrant, so eight trays (Figure 13.3)
- have buccal tubes welded to accommodate both arch wire and headgear (Figure 13.4)
- have size and quadrant etched onto the surface of each band for identification
- have a straight occlusal edge, the gingival edge is contoured
- are for single use only

FIXED APPLIANCES – WHAT THEY DO AND WHAT IS USED

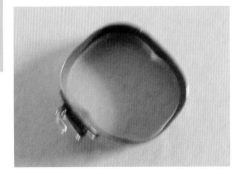

Figure 13.2 Molar band.

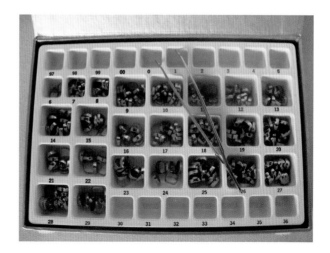

Figure 13.3 Tray of first molar bands.

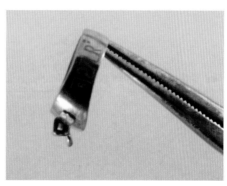

Figure 13.4 Molar band with tube.

(However, if a patient's band comes loose, it can be re-cemented for them but not used for another patient.)

If the molar bands are to be used as part of a trans palatal or lingual arch system, the bands will be soldered to the arch. The other teeth in the arch anterior to the first molars are fitted with brackets. This allows the arch wire which fits into the bracket slots to continue further back into a buccal tube which is attached to the side of the band. There are a great many variations on the size and type of buccal tube that can be used.

Bands can:

- have a variety of auxiliaries:
  - single tubes
  - double tubes
  - triple tubes (Figure 13.5)
- have cleats welded to them, palatally or lingually
- can have triple tubes if two arch wires are being used and headgear (EOT) can also be fitted

FIXED APPLIANCES – WHAT THEY DO AND WHAT IS USED

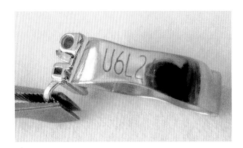

Figure 13.5 Band with triple tube (for EOT).

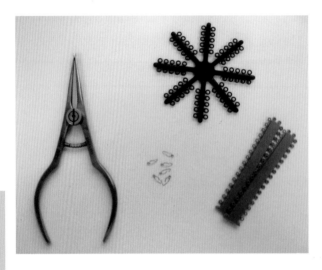

Figure 13.6 Green anterior and blue posterior separating rings, separating springs and separating pliers.

Separation

Bands cannot be fitted in cases of crowding and tight contact points unless the patient has worn separating modules to create an interproximal space to allow the band to be seated comfortably and accurately. These are fitted several days prior to the band fitting to open the contact point. They are placed between the teeth using separating pliers. Springs are occasionally used, placed by pliers, especially for partially erupted teeth (Figure 13.6).

Brackets

They can be made of

- metal (Figure 13.7a):
  - stainless steel
  - are the most commonly used in the growing patient, are tooth-friendly, not as hard as ceramic brackets not likely to fracture with a direct blow (sports, etc.)

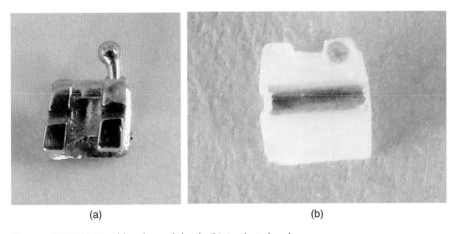

(a)   (b)

Figure 13.7 (a) Metal bracket with hook. (b) Aesthetic bracket.

- aesthetic (Figure 13.7b):
  - tooth coloured or clear
  - not as noticeable
  - superior aesthetics
  - preferred by adults
  - often have metal insert in the arch wire slot as metal slides well over metal which results in less friction and more efficient movement of teeth
  - slightly bulkier

Brackets can be:

- fixed to the labial and buccal surfaces of the teeth. This is more easily accessible for the clinician but is visible
- fixed to the lingual (palatal and tongue) surfaces of the teeth, when it is not visible
- self-ligating or conventional requiring the arch wire to be held into the bracket with ligatures or O-rings

They have a rectangular section channel (slot) in the bracket which houses the arch wire. Round section wires do not fit as snugly as rectangular wires. This allows some 'play' while rectangular wires are more firmly engaged.

- Brackets are almost always of the pre-adjusted design
- The prescription dictates the levels of tip and torque
- (torque is the correction of inclination labiolingually)
- These can be to different prescriptions, e.g. Roth, Andrews and MBT
- Each tooth has its own prescribed individual bracket
- Pre-adjusted brackets developed from the Begg technique are marketed as the Tip Edge system

FIXED APPLIANCES – WHAT THEY DO AND WHAT IS USED

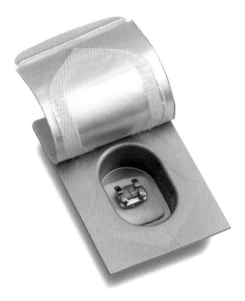

The arch wire is held positively in the bracket by:

- a metal ligature

or

- an elastomeric

Some self-ligating brackets do not use this method

- they have a latch built into the bracket itself, which makes it self-ligating
- the latch is opened to insert or remove the arch wire using a special tool that opens and closes the latch

Brackets can either be

- fixed to the tooth by applying composite adhesive in the surgery
- come from the manufacturer ready pre-coated with adhesive (Figure 13.8)

There are two techniques for doing this:

- Direct bonding – fixing the individual attachments directly onto the teeth (most commonly used)
- Indirect bonding – positioning them on a model, transferring them to a tray, placing tray in mouth and curing them together through it

It is crucial that the brackets are placed very accurately, because if they are at the wrong height or angulation the tooth will not subsequently align correctly.

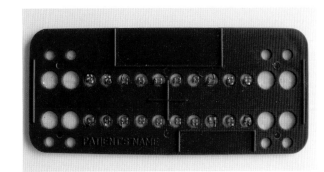

Figure 13.9 Metal brackets on orientation card.

Brackets are:

- usually mounted on orientation cards for ease of delivery (Figure 13.9)
- often have a coloured identification dot to show which way up they are and for which tooth
- some have angles of torque as well as tip built into the wire slot
- popular prescriptions are Roth, Andrews and MBT (McLauglin, Bennett and Trevisi)
- canine brackets can have 'hooks' to aid elastic wear
- osteotomy patients often need hooks on canines and premolars
- bases are textured for extra glue retention
- are contoured to the surface of the tooth

Very occasionally a Begg bracket is used as single attachments together with a removable appliance which uses a whip arm spring to extrude or intrude a tooth.

Brackets can be supplied with gold chain attached to them (These are fitted in theatre under general anaesthesia when patients are having ectopic canines exposed).

Buccal tubes

Buccal tubes are an attachment in their own right (Figure 13.10).

They can be used when the fixed appliance does not need to include molar bands.

All attachments are bonded.

The buccal tube can come with or without a hook. The hook is placed towards the gingival as opposed to the occlusal part of the tooth. The direction of the hook is towards the back of the mouth, i.e. the 'open' end faces distally.

FIXED APPLIANCES – WHAT THEY DO AND WHAT IS USED

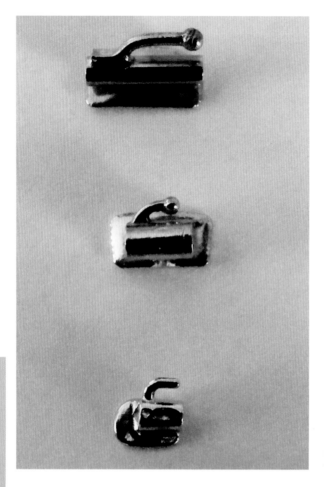

Figure 13.10 Buccal tubes.

This hook has a function similar to a hook which forms part of a bracket or a crimpable hook that is fixed onto an arch wire. It can be used as a point to attach inter- or intra-maxillary elastics.

Buccal tubes:

- can be used both instead of and in addition to molar bands
- that is, on first and second molars
- can also come pre-coated with adhesives

Eyelets, cleats and buttons

Extra attachments that can be bonded onto molar or other teeth to provide traction points (Figures 13.11 and 13.12).

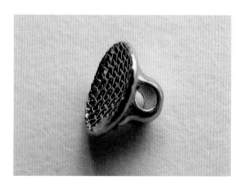

Figure 13.11 Eyelet.

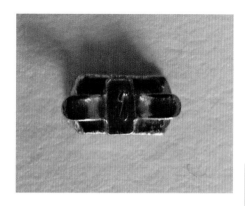

Figure 13.12 Cleat.

ARCH WIRES

They come in various sizes and fit into the channel in the bracket, known as the slot. Initially, a very flexible fine arch wire is placed that causes the teeth to move into alignment. Later, in heavier, more rigid wires the teeth can also be moved along the arch wire.

Each orthodontist has their own preferred sequence of wire changes.

There are several materials from which wires are made:

- stainless steel (SS) (Figure 13.13)
- nickel titanium (NiTi)
- copper NiTi
- beta titanium

They come in various cross sections:

- round
- rectangular
- multi-stranded or braided, e.g. twist flex

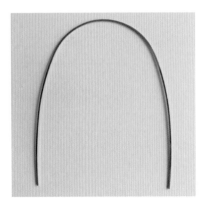

Figure 13.13 Stainless steel arch wire.

are supplied:

- pre-formed for upper and lower arches in a variety of shapes either individually wrapped or in packets
- SS, NiTi, and beta titanium, round and rectangular
- on spools, the length is cut off as required
- in tubes, cut to length (mono filament, braided, co-axial, stranded wire)

The thickness (gauge) of wire governs the amount of force being used.

These range from very light to heavy wires.

When they are fully engaged in the bracket slots and ligated or 'O-ringed' in, the force is then applied onto the tooth.

When force is exerted by using auxiliaries such as springs or elastics, the arch wire is usually passive.

When the teeth are well out of alignment, loops can be bent into the narrow gauge stainless steel arch wire to give greater flexibility and speed up their movement.

Co-axial wire

Have strands of wire wound around a core strand of wire

Twist flex:

- Has three strands of wire wound together (e.g. popular as Wild Cat Wire)

Braided wire:

- Has eight strands of wire formed into a rectangular section wire

Beta Titanium wire:

- can be formed into loops or bends
- is more flexible than SS
- is stronger than NiTi
- is nickel free

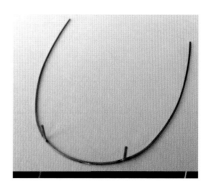

Figure 13.14 Posted arch wire.

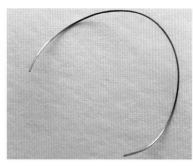

Figure 13.15 Reverse curve arch wire.

Gold coated:

- These are also available for patients with a nickel allergy in both round and rectangular sections

Tooth coloured:

- Aesthetic wires in round and rectangular section (are coated with a tooth coloured plastic material)

Posted wires (Figure 13.14):

- These SS arch wires have posts soldered to them to help when using traction, e.g. to close space
- These posts can be shaped
- The sizes are measured in millimetres between the posts along the anterior curve of the arch wire
- The upper wires range from 30 to 44mm
- The lower wire from 24 to 28mm
- The wires are of rectangular section, usually 0.016″ × 0.022″, 0.018″ × 0.025″ or 0.019″ × 0.025″

Reverse curve wire:

- These wires, known as reverse curve wires (Figure 13.15), which when put on a flat surface 'rock', hence, are not able to be stored in a conventional rack.

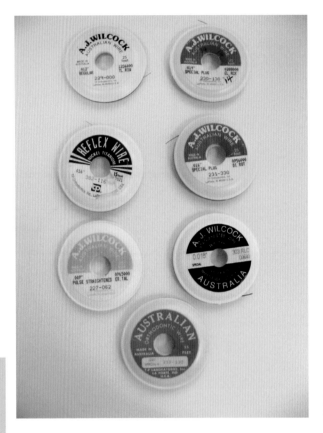

Figure 13.16 Australian wires.

These are inserted to:

- extrude teeth (mid arch)
- reduce an increase of overbite
- and open the bite

Australian wire (Figure 13.16)
This round section wire:

- comes in either 10-inch lengths or spools of 25 feet
- is used with the Begg system, a light wire technique
- is cut as required
- is also popular when making bespoke arch wires with bends and loops
- is supplied in several grades depending on what properties are needed, Regular, Regular Plus, Special and Special Plus to fabricate the individual wire required

Heat activated wires

- Many wires are now available as thermal wires
- They become activated at body heat

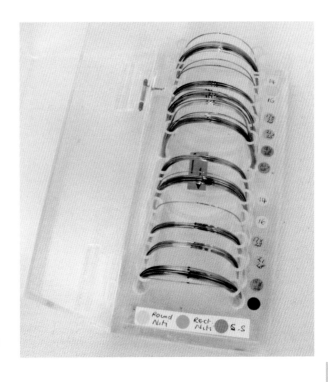

Figure 13.17 Arch wire storage.

Arch wire storage (Figure 13.17)

- Arch wires are kept in covered racks so that they are easily accessible
- In order to mark an arch wire, chinagraph pencils can be used. Due to cross-contamination issues, single-use disposable markers are now used

Lingual arch wires

- Come in Stainless steel, NiTi, Beta Titanium and thermal wires, shaped for lingual anatomy and to accommodate narrow inter bracket dimensions

PLIERS

There are a great many pliers available for use with fixed appliance therapy.

Just as every clinician has their own favoured method of working, they also have their preferred pliers and hand instruments.

Frequently used pliers include:

- Safety hold Flush cut Distal end cutters (for trimming the end of arch wire in the mouth)
- Weingart pliers
- Pin and ligature cutters (for soft and narrow gauge wire)

- Light wire pliers
- Mathieus
- Mosquito forceps
- Crown and band contouring pliers
- Bird beak pliers
- Coon's pliers (for tying ligatures)
- Step pliers (for making 'steps' in the wire, up or down)
- Tweed pliers (rectangular arch forming)
- Tweed loop forming pliers
- Hook crimping pliers
- NiTi cinch back pliers (to turn over the distal end of the arch wire)
- Bracket removing pliers
- Posterior band removing pliers
- Band slitter pliers
- Adhesive removing pliers
- Separating module pliers

However, if you had too many of these on a tray it would be:

- cluttered
- heavy
- require a lot of instruments
- a lot of sterilising capability

So, there are usually between four and six pliers per tray set-up, unless a specific treatment at a certain appointment calls for extra ones.

HAND INSTRUMENTS

In addition to pliers, there are several hand instruments needed. Again, some are common to all procedures, others for specific uses only, such as fitting bands and brackets. Even if they are not normally needed, they must all be available and accessible in case of unforeseen treatment, e.g. breakages.

These include (Figure 13.18):

- ligature director
- plugger
- bite stick
- Mershon band pusher
- College tweezers
- mouth mirror
- probe
- spatula

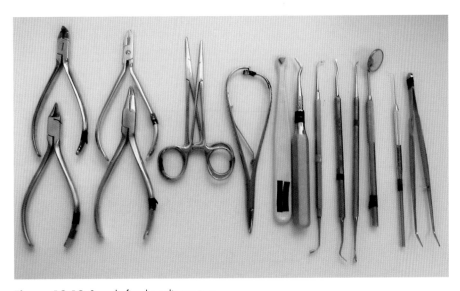

Figure 13.18 Sample fixed appliance tray.

- Mitchell trimmer
- Wards carver
- flat plastic
- Twirl-on (for placing o-rings)
- Mathieu hemostat
- Mosquito hemostat
- Keat and buccal tube tweezers
- direct bonding tweezers, straight or curved
- direct bonding tweezers with bracket aligner
- contra-angled handpieces and debonding burs
- direct bonding adhesive removing pliers

AUXILIARIES

These are the items that are used in addition to bands, brackets and wires in the course of adjusting fixed orthodontic appliances (Figure 13.19a and b).
They include:

- Ligatures:
  - these can be in several thicknesses
  - they can be pre-formed or open
  - a long ligature can be wound across many teeth over the wire as an alternative to O rings

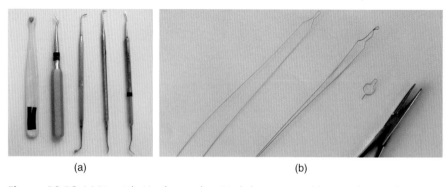

| (a) | (b) |

Figure 13.19 (a) Bite stick, Mershon pusher, Mitchels trimmer and ligature director. (b) Ligature, Kobyashi ligature, 'quick lig' and mosquito.

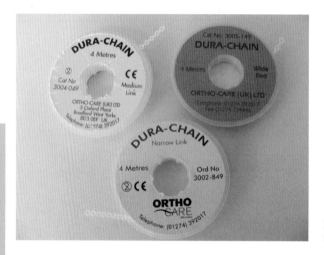

Figure 13.20 Narrow, medium and wide chain.

- can be placed to bridge a span to help support the arch wire
- can be used across many teeth **under** the wire to retain them, e.g. when they are not to be moved. This is known as a lace up
- individual short pre-formed ligatures (quick ligs) can also be used to hold an arch wire securely in a bracket
- often used when greater strength is needed than an 'O'-ring, e.g. severely rotated teeth
- sometimes, can be placed when a hook is needed, e.g. to attach elastics
- this would be a Kobyashi hook, which is a modified ligature (Surgical osteotomy patients, in addition to crimpable hooks and hooks on brackets can have many 'Kobys' in place when they go to theatre to allow for multiple elastic placements both at the time of and post surgery)
- elastic module chain (Figure 13.20)
- supplied on reels, either closed, short or openly spaced

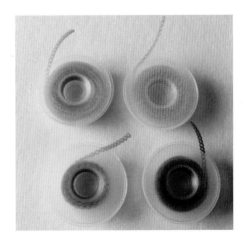

Figure 13.21 Coloured chain.

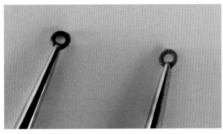

Figure 13.22 Elastomerics in mosquitos.

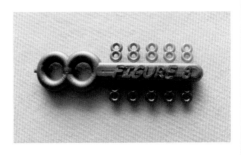

Figure 13.23 Figure-of-eight elastomerics.

- clear, grey or can be coloured (Figure 13.21)
- is used to apply force, e.g. for space closure and lasts sufficiently between appointments

Elastomeric modules (O-rings) (Figure 13.22):

- are used around the bracket to keep the arch wire securely held
- are changed at each visit and at arch wire adjustments
- are put in place with Mathieu pliers or mosquito forceps
- are often tied in 'figure-of-eight' for extra hold, some sold in that shape (Figure 13.23)
- can be clear, white or black and a wide range of colours (Figure 13.24)

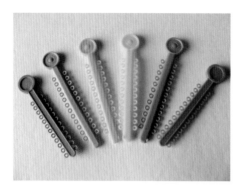

Figure 13.24 Range of coloured O-rings.

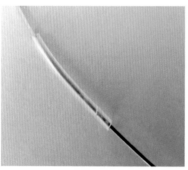

Figure 13.25 Arch wire with sleeving.

Protective sleeving (Figure 13.25):

- is placed over the arch wire where there
- is a large space, e.g. an extraction site to protect the inside of lip or cheek
- protective – useful for patients playing a musical instrument by mouth
- lip bumper (Figure 13.26) – protects soft tissues, easy to fit and remove
- Elastic string
- used to draw teeth together, comes in several strengths, e.g. Zing string

Rotation wedges (Figure 13.27):

- small rubber wedges, fitted under the arch wire and attached under the tie wings of the bracket for rotating teeth
- E-link modules (Figure 13.28) connect brackets 'hook to hook' to rotate individual teeth
- come in variety of sizes

NiTi power springs (Figure 13.29):

- can be used for opening and closing space
- are comfortable for patients
- provide a sustained force
- easier to keep clean, so aids oral hygiene
- reduce the frequency of visits

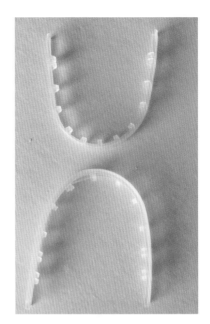

Figure 13.26 Protective bumper which fits over fixed appliance brackets.

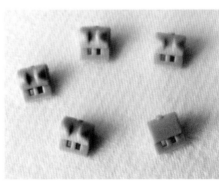

Figure 13.27 Rotation wedges.

Coil (Figure 13.30):

- supplied in spools
  open
  closed
- is cut off to the length required
- arch wire is threaded through coil and is
- activated to open a space
- passive to prevent a space from closing

Intra-maxillary elastics (Figure 13.31):

- are fitted to attachments
- are worn vertically between the upper and lower arch
- are of varying strengths

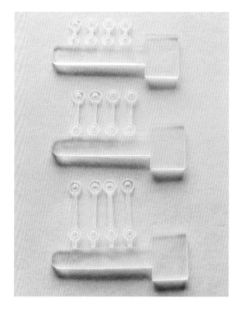

Figure 13.28 Space closing modules.

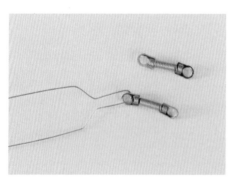

Figure 13.29 Niti power springs.

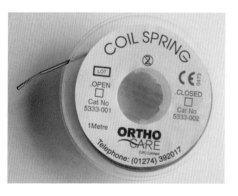

Figure 13.30 Coil.

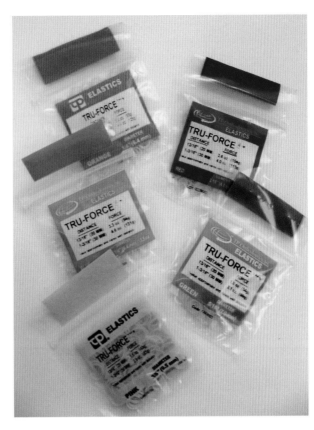

Figure 13.31
Intra-maxillary elastics.

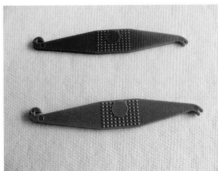

Figure 13.32 Elastic placer.

Elastic placer (Figure 13.32):

- with hooks at each end, this helps patients to fit and remove their elastic bands

Separating modules (Figure 13.33):

- come in two sizes – small for anterior placement, large for posterior
- are smooth, often radiopaque

FIXED APPLIANCES – WHAT THEY DO
AND WHAT IS USED

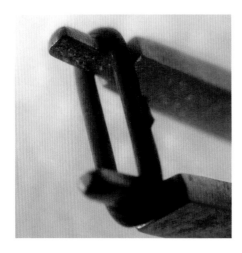

Figure 13.33 Separating module on plier.

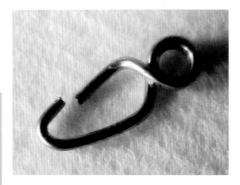

Figure 13.34 Separating spring.

- are placed between teeth some days prior to fitting bands
- separating springs not commonly used now (Figure 13.34), are useful for partially erupted teeth
- are made of metal
- are curved, designed to spring contact points apart
- are fitted between teeth, using pliers

A FIXED APPLIANCE TRAY

For the nurse, it is helpful to have a standard 'tray set-up'
These trays can be made up prior to a clinical session which saves time.
The tray is made up of the instruments that the clinicians like and routinely uses.

FIXED APPLIANCES – WHAT THEY DO AND WHAT IS USED

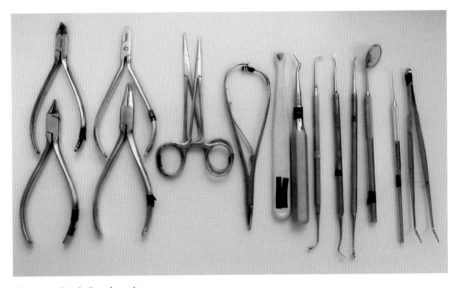

Figure 13.18 Fixed appliance tray.

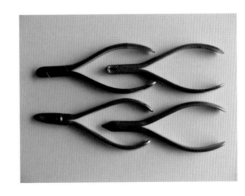

Figure 13.35 Selection of pliers.

A fixed appliance tray (Figure 13.18) set-up might typically include:

- **pliers**
- a pair of:
  - light wire cutters, for cutting soft wire and ligatures
  - distal end cutters, for cutting off excess arch wire behind the molars
  - Weingarts Utility pliers
  - light wire pliers, for loops, cinching, etc.
  - Mosquito forceps
  - Mathieus for placing elastomerics, ligating and tying in (Figure 13.35)

Hand instruments such as:

- Mirror, probe and College tweezers
- Mitchell trimmers – to locate brackets, remove adhesive, etc.

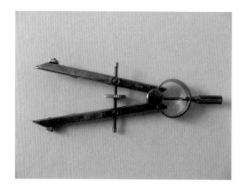

Figure 13.36 Dividers.

- Merton pusher/plugger – to seat and contour molar bands
- Bite stick – to seat bands
- Director/Ligature tucker – to hold wire securely in bracket slot when ligating and to turn under the 'pigtail' of excess wire
- Dividers/rulers (Figure 13.36) – to measure widths between teeth or across the dental arch

are popular choices.

It is necessary, and many orthodontists consider it vital, that they have each patient's study models available for every appointment.

When preparing to adjust a fixed appliance, it is always wise to have everything ready to:

- replace a lost bracket
- re-cement a loose band

Therefore, you always need to have at hand

- the light source
- adhesive
- cements

The orthodontic patient will sometimes present with a breakage which they do not know about.

Always have everything ready for every eventuality.

Keep all the auxiliaries covered and within easy reach.

Have the covered arch wire stands nearby.

Have the light-emitting diode curing light always ready and charged (Figure 13.37).

If extra items are needed, always change gloves before going into drawers, etc.

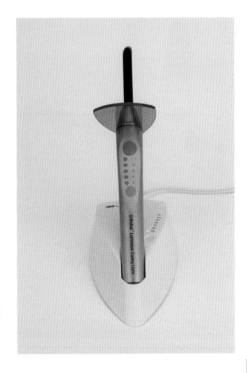

Figure 13.37 Ortholux™ luminous curing light. (Reproduced with permission of 3M Unitek. © 2010 3M Unitek. All rights reserved.)

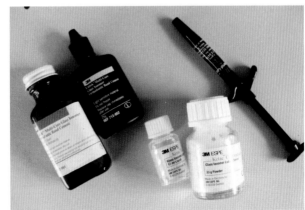

Figure 13.38 Cements. (Reproduced with permission of 3M Unitek. © 2010 3M Unitek. All rights reserved.)

FIXED APPLIANCES – WHAT THEY DO AND WHAT IS USED

CEMENTS

There are several cements that are widely used in orthodontics (Figure 13.38):

- many leach fluoride
- some are powder and liquid mixed and which set in time in the mouth
- some are powder and liquid which is light cured in the mouth

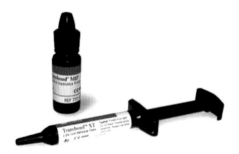

Figure 13.39 Transbond™ XT light cure adhesive. (Reproduced with permission of 3M Unitek. © 2010 3M Unitek. All rights reserved.)

ADHESIVES

There are many orthodontic adhesives on the market of which one is illustrated (Figure 13.39).

- some are ready mixed, dispensed straight from a syringe, light cured
- some are in two parts which need to be mixed together, e.g. base and catalyst
- some leach fluoride
- there are some especially for use in bonding fixed retainers. These tend to flow more easily

If using light cure adhesive when attaching clear brackets, the working time is reduced as the heat and light from the operating light will make it set more quickly whereas metal brackets have to have the light applied to them from the side.

ETCHANT/PRIMER

Before fixing the bracket to the tooth, the enamel tooth surface must be prepared.

This can be achieved by:

- washing with acid etch, then drying the tooth and applying primer
- using a system where this process is combined in a single application
- this is known as self-etch primer (SEP) (Figure 13.40)
  (Single doses are available as 'lollipops'. This system does not necessarily need a totally dry field.)

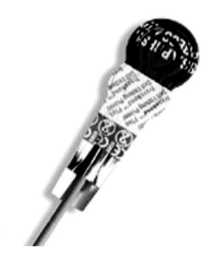

Figure 13.40 Transbond™ plus self-etching primer. (Reproduced with permission of 3M Unitek. © 2010 3M Unitek. All rights reserved.)

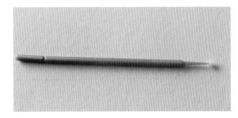

Figure 13.41 Microbrush.

MICROBRUSHES

Microbrushes (Figure 13.41):

- come in a variety of applicator sizes.
- useful when applying etchant or primer to teeth
- disposable

LIP RETRACTORS

Lip retractors (Figure 13.42):

- are usually double-ended, come in small, teenage and large sizes
- can be plastic or metal
- can be used when taking intra-oral photographs
- should be autoclavable

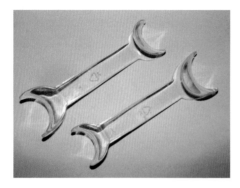

Figure 13.42 Lip retractors.

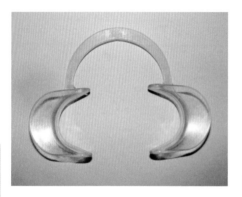

Figure 13.43 Cheek retractors.

CHEEK RETRACTORS

Cheek retractors (Figure 13.43) are:

- all in one piece
- made of plastic
- used to keep the cheeks and lips away from the teeth when bonding
- should be autoclavable

AIDS TO PATIENT COMFORT

Relief wax (Figure 13.44):

- comes in small boxes for patients to self-administer if the appliance is rubbing the inside of the lip/cheek

FIXED APPLIANCES – WHAT THEY DO AND WHAT IS USED

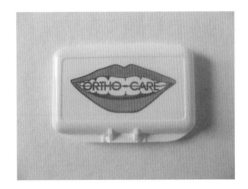

Figure 13.44 Relief wax.

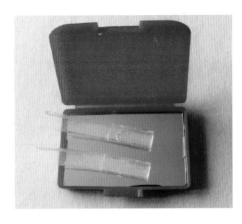

Figure 13.45 Relief silicone.

Silicone (medical grade) (Figure 13.45):

- stays in place more easily
- does not become brittle
- can be used to cover a larger area
- has no taste or smell
- unlike wax, it is not affected by heat

Mouth gel:

- topical application for painful ulcers and abrasions
- quickly removes discomfort
- guards against infection
- must be non-salicylate containing gel (for children)

As there are so many sharp wires and metal bands and brackets associated with these appointments, you must have a sharps bin nearby. You must know and be familiar with the appropriate policy to follow.

With what must seem an alarming array of equipment and consumables around you, it is time to start work.

Every nurse has their own method of working and organisation to keep one step ahead – anticipation is your third hand!

It saves so much time and makes the day run more smoothly.

Chapter 14

Fixed appliances – direct bonding

There are two methods of fitting fixed appliances:

- direct bonding
- indirect bonding

Direct bonding is the more routinely used technique and this chapter aims to highlight the nurse's role in this process.
Different clinicians work in different ways.

- Some clinicians like to work 'four-handed' with a nurse
  - *This means that the nurse hands them the correct instrument at the appropriate time*
  - *Nurses also cut and hand them ligatures, chain, coil, etc.*
  - **This places the tray on the nurse's side**
- Some clinicians prefer to work from the tray themselves
  - They work without the nurse's direct help
  - *They may ask for chain, elastic sleeving, etc. (sometimes cut it themselves)*
  - *The nurse hands a new arch wire*
  - *The clinician often hands the nurse Mathieus, mosquitos, Twirl-ons, etc., whichever they use, for loading O-rings*
  - **This places the tray on the clinician's side**

NB: It is important that at all appointments the patient's model box is available with the study models within reach. Models should be taken out of the box before the treatment begins and the nurse puts on gloves.

COMMUNICATION

Nurses also communicate with and monitor the patient:

- *ask them how they are*
- *ask them what's going on in their life, etc.*
- *ask them what colours of O-rings they want*

while the orthodontist refreshes their own memory reading or writing up the notes, etc.

If the patient is sitting in silence, they are less likely to be brave enough to mention:

- *any concerns or problems they may have about their treatment or appliance*
- *any teasing that they may be experiencing*
- *that they have forgotten the rules, and have a breakage*

ALLERGY AWARENESS

Orthodontic fixed appliance brackets are of stainless steel which can contain nickel, chromium and cobalt. Arch wires are also of stainless steel and nickel-titanium. It is important that any allergy to nickel should be recorded as part of the general medical history and clearly marked on the notes.

ORAL PIERCING

It has become very fashionable for patients to have oral piercings. These can vary:

- from a discreet stud in the lip
- to one or more large lip rings
- through to unilateral or bilateral tongue studs

The patient may or may not be asked to remove these during treatment.

The patient may not able to do this without using a mirror to take it out and replace it.

Patients need to be advised:

- that there is a chance their metal jewellery might damage the appliance, e.g. if it is 'clicked' against a palatal arch
- that the metal might damage the teeth, especially the incisal edges
- that the metal might sit in space closure sites
- that if sharp, the jewellery might puncture the clinician's glove

LOCAL ANAESTHETIC

Local anaesthetic delivered by syringe is very rarely needed when fitting or adjusting appliances.

Topical anaesthetic can be used if required.

FIXED APPLIANCES – DIRECT BONDING

FITTING A FIXED APPLIANCE USING THE DIRECT BONDING TECHNIQUE

The patient has the molar bands and the brackets fitted onto each tooth individually.

This can be done in four ways and depends on:

- the preferences of the clinician
- the age and capabilities of the patient
- fitting times in and around any dental extractions that are required

Method 1

- The patient comes in to have the separators placed
- At the next visit, these are removed and the bands fitted and cemented
- At the third visit, the brackets are bonded

Method 2

- The patient comes in to have the separators placed
- A week later, they have the bands and brackets fitted in one visit

Method 3

- The patient has the separators fitted at the same visit as the brackets
- At the next appointment, they have the separators removed and the bands fitted and cemented

Method 4

- The patient has upper and lower brackets, but with buccal tubes bonded on all first molars instead of molar bands fitted on a single visit

In cases where the patient is planned to have orthognathic surgery, bands are fitted to the first (and usually) second molars

In these patients, hooks can be incorporated into the brackets (Figure 14.1) on canine and premolar teeth. Some clinicians prefer to fit crimpable hooks directly onto the arch wire prior to surgery

NB: When fitting brackets with composite adhesive material, a light source is used.

FIXED APPLIANCES – DIRECT BONDING

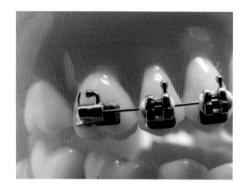

Figure 14.1 Hooks on brackets.

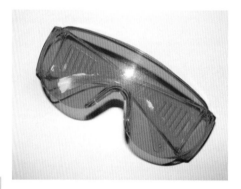

Figure 14.2 Safety glasses for use with light-emitting diode light.

It is important that the patient, orthodontist and nurse wear protective glasses (Figure 14.2) that have orange tinted lenses at all times when they are curing bracket adhesive. No one must look directly at the blue light. Parents in the surgery must either be asked to sit in the waiting room or to look away whilst curing takes place.

METHOD 1 – THREE VISITS

First appointment – putting in the separators

The nurse needs to prepare:

- *the patient's clinical notes*
- *mouth mirror*
- *elastomeric separators*
- *separator placement pliers (Figure 14.3)*
- *floss*
- *a follow-up appointment*

FIXED APPLIANCES – DIRECT BONDING

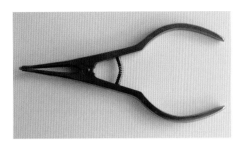

Figure 14.3 Separating pliers.

Procedure

The nurse:

- *ensures that the patient and staff have appropriate personal protection*
- *makes sure that the patient is seated comfortably*
- *establishes which teeth are to be banded at the next visit, as this indicates how many separators are needed*
- *gives the clinician the separators of their choice, loaded on pliers*
- *after they are placed, explains to the patient that:*
  - *separators may feel strange, like a piece of food has become wedged between their teeth*
  - *this feeling will go after a few hours but they may feel some discomfort on these teeth for a day or two*
  - *they cannot use floss in the molar areas while separators are in position*
  - *they will do no harm should they be accidentally swallowed*

Second appointment – fitting and cementing the bands

The nurse will need to prepare:

- *the patient's clinical notes*
- *the model box*
- *mirror, probe and College tweezers*
- *prophylactic handpiece*
- *orthodontic prophylactic paste (oil-free) (Figure 14.4)*
- *rubber cup*
- *dental floss*
- *3-in-1 syringe*
- *suction*
- *cheek retractors*
- *cotton rolls*
- *cement, pad and spatula*
- *box of bands (Figure 14.5) and spare College tweezers*

FIXED APPLIANCES – DIRECT BONDING

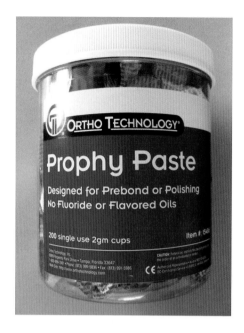

Figure 14.4 Orthodontic prophylactic paste.

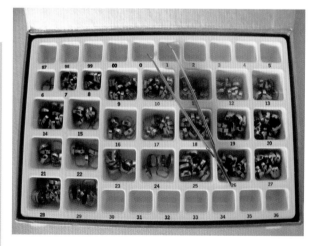

Figure 14.5 Box containing a selection of bands.

- *posterior band remover*
- *Mershon pusher (Figure 14.6)*
- *plugger*
- *bite stick*
- *Mitchell trimmer*
- *patient relief wax or medical-grade silicone*
- *hand mirror*

FIXED APPLIANCES – DIRECT BONDING

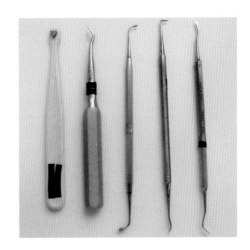

Figure 14.6 Bite stick, Mershon pusher, plugger, Mitchell trimmer and ligature director.

Procedure

- *The nurse ensures that:*
  - *the patient and staff are using personal protective equipment*
  - *the patient is sitting comfortably in the chair. This is a longer appointment and younger patients can get restless and fidgety*
- *Give the clinician a probe so that the separators can be removed*
- The teeth are then flossed
- With a contra-angled handpiece, rubber cup and oil-free prophylactic paste, clean around all the areas that are being treated
- *Get the patient to rinse thoroughly or irrigate the mouth and aspirate*
- Using the study model as a guide for sizing, the clinician chooses the right size molar bands for the teeth in question (these may be first molars, second molars or both)
- *Write down the size of each band to be recorded in the notes*
- Using posterior band removing pliers, remove the bands and dry them
- Ensure that there is a dry field in the mouth, plenty of cotton rolls
- *Mix the cement and line each band with it*
- *Hand them individually to the clinician, with a Mershon pusher, plugger or bite stick, whichever is needed*
- The clinician will then seat the bands on the teeth
- Quickly wipe excess cement away with gauze or cotton wool roll, or leave until nearly set and remove using a Mitchell trimmer
- *Give two damp cotton rolls for the patient to bite down onto until the cement sets*
- With a Mitchell trimmer trim off any flash (excess cement)
- *The patient is then asked to rinse again*
- *Give the patient the hand mirror to see what the brace looks like and ask them to check that there is nothing sharp or uncomfortable*

FIXED APPLIANCES – DIRECT BONDING

- *Give oral hygiene and dietary instructions plus a box of wax or medical-grade silicone, in case the patient has any problems with the appliance rubbing. The cheeks and tongue soon become accustomed to the new appliance*
- *The patient also gets a leaflet, the appliance is explained to them again, and they are reminded what is to be done at the next appointment*

Third appointment – fitting the brackets and arch wires

The patient has the molar bands in place, so the brackets are now fitted. (In adult patients where there are anterior crowns or veneers, it is sometimes necessary to use porcelain primer before bonding brackets to these teeth.)

The nurse needs to prepare:

- *the patient's clinical notes*
- *the model box*
- *mirror probe and College tweezers (Figure 14.7)*
- *prophy handpiece*
- *rubber cups*
- *orthodontic oil-free prophy paste*
- *3-in-1 tips syringe*
- *saliva ejector*
- *light-emitting diode curing light*
- *safety glasses for clinicians, nurses and patient*
- *hand-held shield (Figure 14.8) and shield for light*

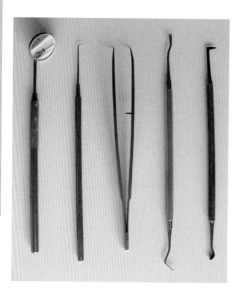

Figure 14.7 Mirror probe, College tweezers, ligature director and Mitchell trimmer.

FIXED APPLIANCES – DIRECT BONDING

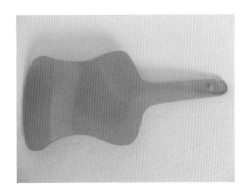

Figure 14.8 Hand-held safety shield.

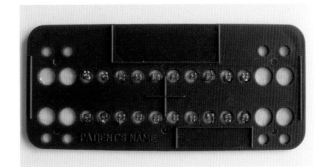

Figure 14.9 Orientation card.

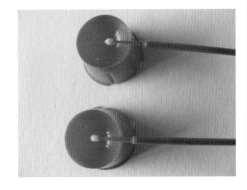

Figure 14.10 Acid etch and primer in Dappen's pots.

- *orientation card (Figure 14.9) of the brackets which are needed*
- *if self-ligating brackets are used, the hand instrument for closing the bracket*
- *cheek retractors*
- *cotton wool rolls*
- *acid etch in disposable Dappen's pot (Figure 14.10) and microbrush*
- *primer in disposable Dappen's pot and microbrush (or self-etch primer (Figure 14.11) in 'lollipop')*
- *light-curing adhesive (syringe or tube) – not needed if using pre-coated brackets*

FIXED APPLIANCES – DIRECT BONDING

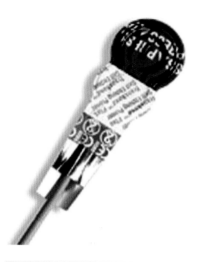

Figure 14.11 Transbond self-etching primer (Reproduced with permission of 3M Unitek. © 2010 3M Unitek. All rights reserved)

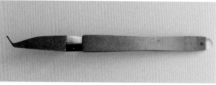

Figure 14.12 Bracket-holding tweezers.

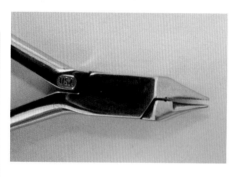

Figure 14.13 205 Light-wire pliers.

- *quick ligs – for tying in individual teeth*
- *bracket-holding tweezers (Figure 14.12)*
- *Mitchell trimmer*
- *light-wire pliers (Figure 14.13)*
- *Weingart pliers (Figure 14.14)*
- *distal-end cutters (Figure 14.16)*
- *Mathieu pliers (Figure 14.17)*
- *mosquito forceps*
- *a selection of initial arch wires*
- *O-rings*
- *bumper-sleeve (if needed, to protect soft tissues adjacent to a wide span of wire)*

FIXED APPLIANCES – DIRECT BONDING

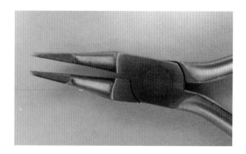

Figure 14.14 Weingart pliers.

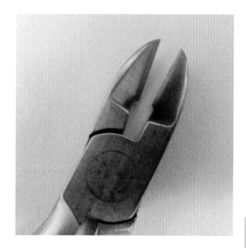

Figure 14.15 Ligature and pin cutter.

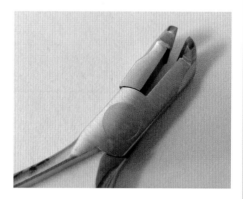

Figure 14.16 Distal-end cutters.

- *sharps box for excess trimmed wire*
- *hand mirror and brushes for oral hygiene instruction*
- *patient's instruction leaflet*
- *box of patient relief wax or medical-grade silicone*

FIXED APPLIANCES – DIRECT BONDING

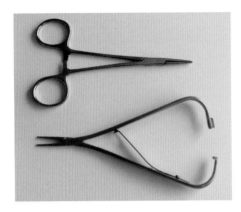

Figure 14.17 Mosquitos and Mathieus.

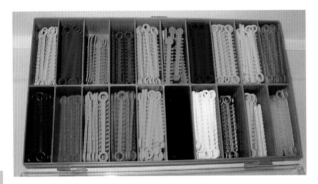

Figure 14.18 Box of coloured O-rings.

Procedure

- *The nurse ensures that patient and staff have the appropriate personal protection*
- *The patient is made comfortable (this is another long visit and for the younger patient it can be hard to sit still)*
- *Show the patient the choice of coloured O-rings (Figure 14.18)(this allows them to customise their appliance)*
- Self-ligating brackets do not need elastomerics or ligatures
- *Check that there have not been any problems since the last visit*
- *Get the brackets on their orientation tray ready*
- *Remove from the tray any brackets not needed, i.e. unerupted or extracted teeth*
- *If the procedure uses the etch and prime method, have etchent and primer in separate disposable Dappen's pots, with microbrushes*
- *If an all-in-one system of self-etch primer is being used, get the 'lollipop' ready*
- With a contra-angled prophylactic handpiece, rubber cup and some oil-free prophylactic paste, clean all the surfaces to be treated
- Wash the teeth thoroughly

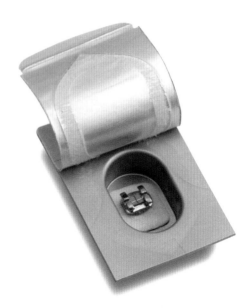

Figure 14.19 VS APC PLUS open blister
(Reproduced with permission of 3M Unitek.
© 2010 3M Unitek. All rights reserved)

- *Allow the patient to either rinse or aspirate*
- A cheek retractor is fitted
- The teeth are isolated and dried thoroughly
- A spot of etchant is placed on the labial surface of each tooth at bracket height
- After a brief period, this is washed off
- *Aspirate and dry again*
- Place a spot of primer onto the labial surface of each tooth at bracket height. *Either*:
  - *load the base of the bracket with adhesive from the syringe*
    or
  - *remove the pre-coated bracket from its protective bubble wrapping (Figure 14.19)*
- *Hand to the clinician on bracket-holding tweezers (when using self-etch primer 'lollipops', once they have been activated and the tip of the micro-brush becomes coated, it 'paints' the solution onto the surface of the tooth and the bracket is positioned)*

Keep doing this until all the brackets have been fitted in the quadrant/arch.

It depends on clinical preference, in which sequence you work and how many brackets are placed before light curing.

Some clinicians cure every bracket individually, others will cure a quadrant, others an entire arch (Figure 14.20).

After all brackets are in position:

- *remove the cheek retractor and let the patient rest a minute (it will feel strange, so a word of encouragement will be helpful)*

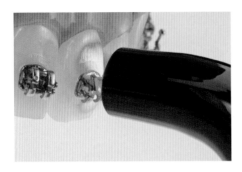

Figure 14.20 Light-curing adhesive on bracket. (Reproduced with permission of 3M Unitek. © 2010 3M Unitek. All rights reserved.)

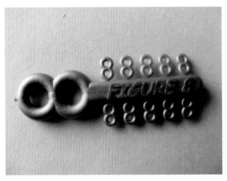

Figure 14.21 Figure-of-eight elastomeric.

- *then an arch wire is selected and cut to just a little longer than the patient's arch length*
- the wire is first fitted into the molar tubes and then eased into the bracket slots
- the chosen O-rings are then placed

As it is the first arch wire, the O-ring is placed over the arch wire, around the outside rim of the bracket under the tie wings.

Later wires might need to be tied in more tightly, so the O-ring is tied in a figure-of-eight (Figure 14.21). Some modules are supplied in this shape and they hold the wire in more tightly.

The distal end cutting pliers are now used to cut off any excess wire distally, that is protruding out of the buccal tube.

If the wire is bendable, then the clinician may choose instead to cinch the wire (that is to turn the end towards the gingiva). This makes it harder for the arch wire to slide out of the tube or to slew around to one side so that one end becomes too long and sticks into the patient's cheek.

- *Check that the patient feels comfortable*
- *Give them oral hygiene instructions, demonstrating the special brushes, etc.*
- *Explain the importance of following dietary advice*
- *Show them how to use the medical-grade silicone or relief wax and give them a box*

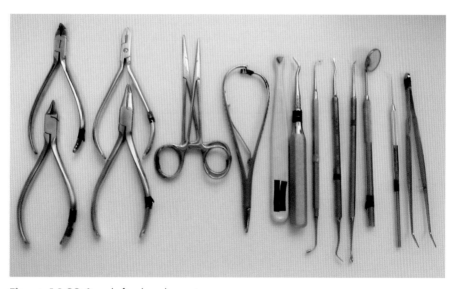

Figure 14.22 Sample fixed appliance tray.

- *Demonstrate how to clean and look after the appliances*
- *Check whether they still have their original leaflet, if not, give them another one*
- *Show them themselves in the mirror*
- *Admire, admire, admire*
- *Tell them they have been a really good patient*

Advise the patient that now the wires are starting to move all the teeth involved in the appliance, there will be some discomfort especially when chewing. Therefore, a soft diet and very small pieces of food are advisable. This may be needed for a few days.

For some children, the first experience of dental treatment is their orthodontics. For them, it is a new experience and can be quite daunting.

Fixed appliance trays (Figure 14.22) have all the equipment that may be needed; sometimes it is not all used but often it is.

METHOD 2 – TWO VISITS

This method has one very brief visit followed by a much longer one:

- separators
- brackets and bands fitted together

This method uses the same layout for the initial separating appointments.

FIXED APPLIANCES – DIRECT BONDING

At the next appointment, the bands and the brackets are fitted at the same appointment. This means all pliers and hand instruments from the bracket and band-fitting procedures must be available.

METHOD 3 – TWO VISITS

- separators and brackets
- bands

At the first appointment, separators are placed, and then the brackets are fitted.

At the second appointment, the separators are removed, the bands fitted and the arch wires placed.

Patients sometimes accidentally lose a bracket; this can be repaired at the second visit.

METHOD 4 – ONE VISIT

- brackets and buccal tubes

This is much the quickest method as there is no need for separation as no bands are fitted.

When the brackets are fitted and buccal tubes fixed to all first molars, this is done in one continuous process. Some clinicians like to place and cure the buccal tubes first. They may do these individually if excess saliva collects.

OTHER USES AND APPLICATIONS FOR FIXED APPLIANCES

Sectional fixed

It is also possible to have:

- small
- localised
- sectional
- single arch

fixed appliances.

These are used if there is a specific isolated problem. It may involve only a few brackets, e.g. uprighting a tipped molar prior to bridgework.

Additional 'piggyback' arch wires

Sometimes, when the arch wire is placed, there is a tooth which is just too far out of alignment for the arch wire to flex into the bracket to be engaged.

When this happens, a small auxiliary wire is used which is placed alongside the main wire. This is known as a piggyback wire and is ligated in with it, but it has the flexibility to engage the outreach tooth into a position which will enable it to be eventually included into the main wire.

PREPARE FOR EVERY EVENTUALITY

Now that their fixed appliance has been fitted and the active phase of treatment has begun, the teeth are on the move.

Between now and the date of debonding, there will be many appointments.

At a routine adjustment appointment you are never quite certain what problems the patient may have before they arrive. Sometimes they themselves do not even know if they have a broken arch wire or a loose bracket.

Prepare for the expected and plan for the unexpected.

In addition to having the routine equipment necessary to adjust fixed appliances, it is helpful to have as much to hand for the unexpected.

In orthodontics, as in most things, as you gain experience over a period of time, you can plan ahead and anticipate what will be needed.

Also, many clinicians are creatures of habit. As the treatment progresses, they have a sequence of arch wires which they favour. They also work in the mouth in an established pattern, e.g. left to right or upper before lower arch.

Getting to know these ways really helps. It keeps the nurse one step ahead and the appointments on track.

FIXED APPLIANCES – DIRECT BONDING

Chapter 15

Fixed appliances – indirect bonding and lingual orthodontics

This chapter is an extension of the two previous ones that dealt with fixed appliances which were directly bonded onto the labial surface of the teeth.

However, attachments can also be bonded onto the teeth using an indirect method. This is a technique that is also frequently used when bonding attachments to the lingual surfaces.

LINGUAL ORTHODONTICS

The Lingual technique is becoming more widely used as patients are increasingly aware of the advantages and possibilities that it makes available.

Many clinicians are now practised in the technique and are able to offer it to their patients. This treatment is an alternative to conventional fixed appliances and are fixed to the labial aspect of their teeth (Figure 15.1).

Lingual orthodontics was initially pioneered in the 1970s in Japan, where it was intended as an alternative for patients who took part in martial arts, and in America, where it was seen as an aesthetic option.

The development was slow as the 1980s saw the introduction of aesthetic brackets and invisible aligners, which offered patients another, less visible, alternative to metal brackets.

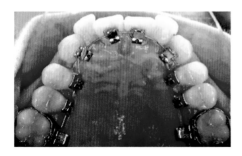

Figure 15.1 Lingual appliance. (Reproduced with permission of Paul Ward, British Lingual Orthodontic Society.)

There has been a renewed interest in lingual orthodontics rather than aligners as an option due to:

- the high laboratory cost of aligners, especially if one gets lost or broken
- they need a high level of patient compliance
- the limited treatments they can provide

Advantages of lingual orthodontics

- of particular benefit to patients who play musical instruments by mouth, especially clarinets and saxophones
- good aesthetic effect especially for adults in occupations where appearance is very important

Disadvantages

- patients sometimes have difficulties with speech
- there can be trauma to edges of the tongue (ulceration)

WHAT MATERIALS ARE USED

Because of their position in the mouth, the pliers and hand instruments that are used to fit and adjust labial appliances would be of little use with lingual appliances. They need to have very fine edges which allow easy access to the brackets and give a less restricted view in the mouth. Impression materials are usually rubber based and models are cast in stone or a hard material.

Brackets

For ease of use, many lingual appliances use self-ligating brackets, but there are systems available which require ligatures or O-rings (Figure 15.2).

Many of these appliances are fitted using the indirect bonding technique but some, notably those which concentrate on the anterior segment only, use direct bonding.

Brackets tend to be smaller, and the bases curved to accommodate the lingual surface.

Wires

The main difference between labial and lingual arch wires is in the shape.

FIXED APPLIANCES – INDIRECT BONDING

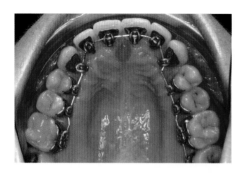

Figure 15.2 Lingual appliance with gold brackets. (Reproduced with permission of Paul Ward, British Lingual Orthodontic Society.)

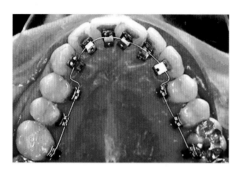

Figure 15.3 Lingual appliance – note shape of arch wire. (Reproduced with permission of Paul Ward, British Lingual Orthodontic Society.)

Lingual arch wires (Figure 15.3) look rather like mushrooms as they have a rounded top, which fits around the anterior teeth and then a 'bend' inwards to accommodate the differing canine/premolar width before flaring to attach to the premolars and molars.

Wires come as upper and lower, and in the same metal as non lingual techniques.

Round wire sizes:

- 010″
- 012″
- 013″
- 014″
- 016″

Square wire sizes:

- 0.016″ × 0.016″
- 0.017″ × 0.017″

Rectangular wire sizes:

- 016″ × 022″
- 017″ × 017″
- 017″ × 025″

FIXED APPLIANCES – INDIRECT BONDING

come in:

- small
- medium
- large

PLIERS

- ligature cutters come in 40°, 50° or 60° of angulation and have reversed or regular curves depending on where they are to be used
- Mathieu pliers are curved
- Weingarts pliers have a 60° angle
- bracket removing pliers and cinch back pliers are of a special design
- distal end cutters must be safety hold

When a patient requires extractions as part of their treatment plan it is usual to have this done a week prior to the fitting of the lingual appliances. When the patient is having a lingual appliance fitted using the indirect technique, the appliance is fitted before the extractions are carried out. The arch wire is removed to allow the dentist access for the extractions. This is to prevent the teeth adjacent to the extraction sites from moving between the time of extraction and fitting of the appliance.

ORAL HYGIENE

Oral hygiene techniques when wearing lingual appliance have many similarities to those used when wearing labial appliances and include:

- a tooth brush
- an interspace (tufted spiral) brush
- wax
- floss
- disclosing tablets
- mouthwash

All are used to help maintain a healthy mouth.

Toothbrush

For the anterior teeth, use the same technique as you would with labial bonding, using a circular motion make the tips of the bristles remove the plaque from the gingival margins towards the occlusal or incisal areas.

FIXED APPLIANCES – INDIRECT BONDING

Interspace brush

The interspace brush is intended for use after the main brushing with the conventional toothbrush. It is meant to go interdentally and is also used to clean between brackets, if the main brush is too big to get into the crevices.

Wax

Sometimes, the brackets or attachments may feel uncomfortable and irritate the tongue. If this happens, either strips of silicone or wax can be used. This gives temporary relief which allows the soft tissues to heal as the irritation is masked. It is best to apply this after brushing the teeth. Using a piece of gauze or some cotton wool make the surface of the bracket as dry as possible. Take a section of wax or silicone and press it over the bracket, this will act like a 'plaster' and make the mouth feel more comfortable.

Floss

Because it is more difficult to reach the brackets, it is helpful to use the long, ready cut lengths of floss which are stiffened at each end and have an area of thick, 'furry' floss in the middle. The stiffened end is threaded under the arch wire and using a 'sawing' action back and forth, it goes inter proximally and under the gingiva and clears any residual plaque.

Disclosing tablets or solution

It is more difficult to see the areas which may be being missed out when brushing, so advise using a disclosing tablet or solution which contains coloured dye. By chewing the tablet, or rinsing with a liquid, the dye mixes with the saliva in the mouth and stains any areas of plaque. This makes it easier to spot and be removed by further brushing. However, the E numbers of some dyes makes people hyper-active, so it is best to check there is no intolerance before suggesting that they are used. Patients may need a mouth mirror to see the lingual surfaces when they look in the bathroom mirror.

Mouthwash

As with labial fixed appliances, it is recommended that the patient uses a fluoride mouth wash every day.

FITTING A LINGUAL APPLIANCE

Lingual appliances are nearly always bonded using the indirect method, with either a chemical cure or light-curing adhesive.

FIXED APPLIANCES – INDIRECT BONDING

THE INDIRECT BONDING TECHNIQUE

While the technique of indirect bonding has been in use for over 25 years, it is the technique of direct bonding onto the labial surface of the tooth that is still more widely used.

However, indirect bonding of fixed appliances is becoming more popular. The patient still has attachments bonded onto their teeth but this uses a different method.

Indirect bonding suffered some problems in the initial stages, which have now largely been overcome as advances in speciality adhesives, transparent thermoplastic trays and customised guidelines for bracket placements have been refined.

It was seen to overcome some of the disadvantages of direct bonding which included:

- difficulty in accessing mal-aligned teeth
- locating precise bracket position might be difficult as hard to see
- attachment may become dislodged and so be incorrectly sited during bonding
- the procedure is clinically time-intensive as only one bracket is positioned at a time
- the younger patients may become restless and fidget

The main difference between the two techniques is that:

- direct bonding involves the clinician precisely placing each bracket on the tooth
- indirect bonding involves all the brackets being incorporated into a transfer tray after accurate placement is made on a model

It is a technique that usually involves the dental technician. The clinician will send the work to be done either to an outside specialist laboratory or to an in-house technician or member of the dental team who has been given training in the technique.

It is important that the clinician fills in a detailed laboratory request form. This must include:

- whether it is for labial or lingual appliances
- for upper or lower or both
- a full arch or a sectional one
- the type of brackets to be used
- information on any teeth not to be bonded
- any over corrections that may be needed
- whether there is to be any interproximal stripping, and if so, where and how much
- which type of bonding trays are needed

FIXED APPLIANCES – INDIRECT BONDING

- vacuum moulded (clear thermoplastic)
- hard acrylic or silicone (if a two tray system is used)

Some technicians use computer programs to calculate the bracket positions on teeth. Others use the work model, and using vertical height and long-axis lines draw a pencil grid on the tooth.

There are several techniques used in indirect bonding. Some methods use a single bonding tray and others use a flexible inner bonding tray with a rigid covering tray over that.

THE ONE BONDING TRAY METHOD USING CHEMICAL CURE ADHESIVE

Prior to the fitting appointment

- the clinician would have taken rubber based impressions of the teeth
- these would go to the laboratory to be cast
- a detailed instruction sheet would be given to the technician
- on the working model, measurements were made to accurately position the bracket on each tooth
- brackets were attached to the teeth on the model
- a thermoplastic tray was made over these
- the tray was removed with the brackets remaining in situ

For the fitting appointment the nurse needs to prepare:

- *clinical notes*
- *the bonding trays and work models*
- *mouth mirror*
- *probe and two pairs of College tweezers*
- *acetone in container*
- *adhesive (in two pots)*
- *frozen holder to keep them as cold as possible*
- *Dappen's pot*
- *microbrushes*
- *sand blasting equipment*
- *etchant*
- *dry field system*
- *3-in-1 tips*
- *cotton wool rolls*
- *pledgets*
- *CA handpiece and rose head burs*
- *scalers*
- *floss*
- *mouthwash and tissues*

- *hand mirror*
- *relief wax or medical grade relief silicone*
- *instruction leaflets*

Procedure at the fitting appointment

- *the nurse ensures that the dentist, patient and nurse have personal protective equipment*
- the clinician tries in and checks the trays
- *the nurse will then clean the trays with acetone*
- the clinician then sandblasts the 'fitting' surfaces of individual teeth
- each tooth takes 3–4 seconds
- *the patient then thoroughly rinses and the nurse aspirates to clear the mouth*
- the clinician attaches a dry field system (if both arches are being treated, the lower arch is done first)
- acid etch is applied and removed after 30 seconds by the clinician, who then inserts cotton wool rolls and dries the mouth and all tooth surfaces
- *at this point, the nurse removes adhesive from the fridge* (as chemical cure adhesive must be kept cool, once removed from fridge)
- *the two containers are placed into the very cold container for the pots*
- *the nurse puts four drops of each fluid in two Dappen's pots, mixing together with a microbrush*
- *the nurse coats the base of the brackets with this solution*
- the clinician paints the surfaces of the teeth
- the tray is inserted firmly and held until the excess solution has set hard, usually in around 3 minutes
- leaving this in place, the procedure may be repeated on the upper teeth
- the trays are then taken out and all residual excess material removed with scalers
- using articulating paper, the occlusion is checked for premature contact points
- arch wires, with ligatures or elastomerics, are placed
- *the patient is given dietary advice and oral hygiene instruction by the nurse*
- *either silicone or relief wax is given to the patient in case of discomfort*

THE TWO-TRAY BONDING TRAY METHOD USING LIGHT-CURED ADHESIVE

Prior to the fitting appointment

- a laboratory request was filled in and sent to the technician along with rubber based impressions of the arch/ arches to be bonded
- the models were cast
- the technician calculated and marked the site of the bracket placement

- a bracket was attached onto each required tooth on the model with adhesive (this adhesive will form a custom-made base for the bracket, so when it is bonded to the tooth, only a small amount of adhesive will be necessary)
- a thermoplastic flexible bonding tray was pressure formed
- a rigid acrylic tray was then made which fitted over the flexible one

For the fitting appointment, the nurse needs to prepare:

- *clinical notes*
- *bonding trays and working models*
- *tray set-up*
- *sandblasting equipment*
- *CA handpiece and pumice/prophylactic paste*
- *rubber cup/ wheel*
- *dry field system for moisture control which incorporates a cheek retractor*
- *light-emitting diode (LED) light*
- *yellow protective glasses and hand-held shield*
- *either self-etch primer (SEP) as a 'lollipop' or etchant and primer in Dappen's pots with separate microbrushes*
- *3-in-1 aspirator tips*
- *adhesive*
- *cotton wool rolls*
- *cotton pledgets*
- *CA handpiece and rose head bur*
- *Miller's articulating forceps*
- *articulating paper*
- *hand mirror*
- *relief wax or medical grade silicone*
- *information and instruction leaflets*

Procedure at the fitting appointment

- *the nurse needs to ensure that the dentist, nurse and patient wear personal protective equipment*
- *that the patient is seated comfortably*
- a moisture control and cheek retraction system is inserted
- (as with all bonding procedures good moisture control is vital)
- arches are usually prepared and fitted one at a time, lowers first
- teeth are cleaned with pumice or prophylactic paste using a CA handpiece and a rubber cup/wheel
- some clinicians also use etchant
- after thorough spraying, the area is dried
- the bases of the brackets are coated with adhesive enhancer
- adhesive is then placed over that
- the etched teeth are coated with sealant

- adhesive is placed into the bracket base
- with both flexible and rigid trays together, they are inserted onto the teeth from the back to the front of the mouth
- use a LED light to set adhesive
  (ensure that protective yellow glasses are worn by all- if there is a parent or accompanying person in the room, they may be asked to go to the waiting room for a few minutes or if they remain, to keep their eyes averted when curing)
- remove the rigid tray
- using a scaler cut and peel away the flexible tray
- after checking that the bracket channels are clear, insert arch wires

If the appliance is placed lingually, the clinician must check that there is no occlusal interference.

If this is so, check with articulating paper held in Miller's forceps and using CA slow handpiece and rose head bur, spot grind high spots

As the use of the indirect bonding technique for both lingual and labial appliances becomes more popular, an increasing number of members of the dental team are extending their skills and training within their units or practices, and now mark the models, position the brackets and construct the bonding tray. Nurses, trained by their clinician, can do the preparation in-house that would previously have been sent to the laboratory. This is only applicable when treating mild cases. This skill opens the way for an extended role for the nurse both in the preparation and fitting of the appliance.

FIXED APPLIANCES – INDIRECT BONDING

Chapter 16

Ectopic canines

Normally, teeth erupt in sequence.

The permanent molars erupt distal to the deciduous dentition.

Incisors, canines and premolar teeth erupt into the space left by the exfoliated deciduous teeth.

An approximate guide to molar eruption is:

- first molars (the 6s) at 6 years
- second molars (the 7s) at 12 years
- third molars (the 8s) between 18 and 25 years (these are often referred to as wisdom teeth)

THE PROBLEM

Eruption is usually straightforward but occasionally a tooth fails to erupt because:

- the root of the baby tooth does not resorb and stays firm
- the permanent tooth is deflected and is late in eruption, or remains unerupted
- the required space is lost and either it stays unerupted, impacted or erupts out of alignment
- the presence of a supernumerary tooth impedes the eruption of a permanent tooth, e.g. upper incisor

If a tooth remains unerupted and out of position, it is said to be ectopic, a specifically diagnostic term for a tooth following an incorrect path of eruption, which may be a reflection of abnormal crypt position or crowding.

This causes problems and the teeth which are most likely to fail to erupt because they are off course are the upper canines (Figure 16.1).

This is more common in females than males.

It is a condition that may have a hereditary factor (can run in families).

The upper canine begins its development high in the maxilla and has a longer distance to travel than any other tooth in the dentition, before it erupts.

More than three quarters of ectopic canines lie palatally to the dental arch.

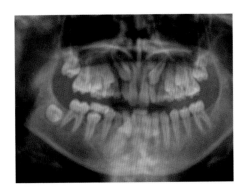

Figure 16.1 Radiograph of ectopic canines.

By about 10 years, there is usually a bulge which can be palpated in the buccal sulcus to indicate that the tooth is on line. If it is not there, then the situation needs to be watched.

The dentist needs to monitor the progress of the tooth. In order to see just where it is and why it may not be erupting, radiograph(s) are taken. This also shows whether the crown of the permanent tooth is impacting into the roots of nearby incisors. This may cause them damage.

While this may be damaging, it is a painless process. Sometimes, the first sign that the ectopic tooth is in contact with and has severely damaged the root of a neighbouring tooth is that the tooth with the damaged root becomes loose. This can happen quite rapidly and may possibly result in the loss of this tooth. Because they are adjacent to the canines, the damaged tooth is often the lateral incisor. The orthodontist needs to know exactly where the unerupted tooth is lying in relation to the adjacent teeth.

It may be either:

- palatal (in the palate)
- labial (on the cheek side of the alveolus)
- across the dental arch (occasionally)

In order to find out the exact position, there is not always sufficient information provided by an orthopantogram alone. A periapical or lateral oblique occlusal of the area may also be needed to precisely locate the position and check on other possible anomalies.

If the canine (the 3) is not severely displaced then the extraction of the retained deciduous canine (the C) may often provide sufficient space to encourage its permanent successor to erupt.

However, these canine teeth sometimes:

- remain unerupted and buried in the maxilla
- erupt into the palate (infrequently)

Ectopic and/or unerupted canines are much rarer in the mandible than the maxilla.

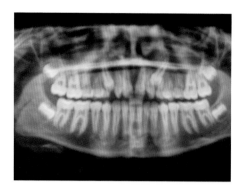

Figure 16.2 Radiograph of bilateral upper ectopic canines in an older child.

Treatment to retrieve these teeth can take many months and the patient has to be cooperative and understand that the treatment will take longer, especially if other features of the malocclusion have to be treated as well.

If a patient has not been referred in at the correct time (approximately 11 years old) and has a retained upper C (Figure 16.2) by the time they are in their mid-teens, they have a dilemma. They may have to:

- leave the baby tooth in situ and wait for it to finally fail
- have it extracted and replaced with a bridge or implant
- have it extracted and seek an orthodontic solution to retrieve the permanent tooth

An orthodontic solution may mean that the patient could still be wearing fixed braces long after their peers have had theirs removed.

If the patient decides to proceed with an orthodontic solution, a treatment plan is made also taking into account other features of the malocclusion.

CLINICAL INTERVENTION – WHAT THE TREATMENT INVOLVES

- A small surgical procedure to expose the buried tooth (this is usually done under general anaesthetic)
- A 'window' is cut in the palatal or buccal soft tissues and any bone over the buried tooth is removed
- A gold-plated eyelet, often with chain (Figure 16.3) or a bracket, is attached to the tooth
- The wound is packed and the site is sutured, with the chain, if fitted, visible

This attachment provides a 'handle' that can be used to attach wire, linked chain, elastic string, etc. to apply traction to begin to gently pull on the tooth.

ECTOPIC CANINES

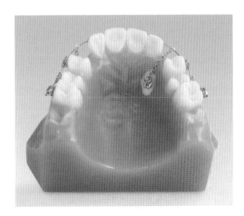

Figure 16.3 Gold eyelet and chain.

This traction is usually applied in conjunction with a fixed appliance on the standing teeth, and after each visit, as the tooth comes near to alignment the number of links of gold chain can be reduced.

Light forces must be used.

Shorter and more frequent appointments are needed to renew the traction.

It sometimes happens that the tooth, once brought into the dental arch, is found to be rotated, e.g. the buccal aspect is facing the palate. This will need to be de-rotated. This can be a slow procedure and the brackets have to be repositioned as the tooth is being de-rotated.

If the patient is not prepared to extend wearing their appliance to allow time for this to be achieved, it is sometimes possible to reach a compromise. By shaping the tooth and adding composite to the palatal surface, the tooth can be disguised to look as if it is the correct way around. This can give a good aesthetic result and is often more acceptable to the patient than several more months of traction to rotate the canine.

If the exposed tooth is lying buccally, then there are two methods of treatment.

- Like the palatal presentation, a fixed appliance can be used
- Less frequently, a removable appliance (Figure 16.4) can be used as a preliminary to a fixed appliance

A metal whip arm (Figure 16.5) from the crib of the removable appliance is positioned at the top (gingival side) of the bracket. This needs to be a correctly placed Begg bracket. The whip puts a force on the bracket and extrudes the tooth.

However, in nearly all cases, fixed appliances are used to retrieve ectopic canines.

ECTOPIC CANINES

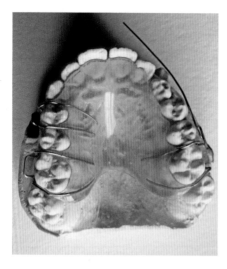

Figure 16.4 Upper removable appliance with untrimmed whip arm.

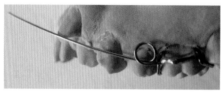

Figure 16.5 Untrimmed whip arm.

The nurse needs to prepare a fixed tray set up:

- *the patient's model box*
- *mirror, probe and College tweezers*
- *light-wire cutters*
- *light-wire pliers*
- *distal-end cutter*
- *Weingart plier*
- *ligature tuckers*
- *Mathieu pliers/mosquito forceps*
- *Coon's ligature locker pliers*
- *ruler*
- *dividers*
- *cheek retractor*
- *topical local anaesthetic, if needed.*
- *3-in-1 tip*
- *fine aspirator tip*

Depending on the preference of the clinician:

- *ligature wire*
- *spool elastic*
- *elastic links (chain)*

- *coil springs*
- *ligatures*
- *elastomerics (O-rings)*
- *cotton wool rolls*
- *Mitchell trimmer*
- *sharps box*
- *arch wire stands*
- *patient relief wax*
- *medical-grade relief silicone*
- *hand mirror*

In some cases, a bracket which is bonded to the exposed canine does not have gold chain attached. *When this happens, it is vital to make sure that the appointment to attach the ligature, elastic or chain is organised for as soon after the surgical pack is removed as possible.* If the soft tissues heal over the exposed tooth, it may prevent access and, in the worst cases, the patient may have to undergo another surgical procedure.

Begg brackets are a popular choice for bonding to the exposed canine and have a vertical channel running through them, which would normally house a Begg pin. This means that the ligature, elastic thread, etc. can easily be threaded straight through this channel.

Where there is difficulty with access or vision, the clinician will sometimes make an eyelet from 0.012″ ligature wire and pass the wire through the bracket channel as an easier way of fixing traction to the bracket.

Procedure

- *The nurse needs to assist the clinician at the chairside to ensure:*
  - *that the patient and clinicians are wearing personal protection*
  - *that the patient is made comfortable*
- A cheek retractor is inserted
- Using a 3-in-1 tip and aspirating, the wound is checked by the clinician to make sure that the pack has been fully removed and the bracket is clear of any obstruction
- *The wound area is prone to bleeding, especially on the first visit when the pack is removed and the nurse must keep the area free from oozing blood and excess saliva (a supply of cotton wool rolls to apply pressure)*
- *If there is a change of arch wire, the new size must be chosen and prepared* (the existing arch wire may be reused)
- *The colour of the O-rings to be used is selected by the patient and prepared by the nurse*
- These are put on using either of the following:
  - Mathieus, which can hold O-rings, twist ligatures, place elastics or chain
  - Coon's pliers, which tie ligatures (not quick ligs)

ECTOPIC CANINES

- - Twirl-ons, a hand instrument which stretches O-rings open to place over the tie wings of a bracket
  - haemostats, which hold O-rings, tie ligatures and quick ligs and can place chain
  - mosquitos, which hold O-rings, tie ligatures and quick ligs and can place chain
- The O-rings on the fixed appliance are removed
- The arch wire is taken out and either adjusted or replaced
- O-rings or ligatures are placed around each bracket, O-rings are often placed in a 'figure-of-eight' pattern for extra retention
- Traction is then applied to the exposed canine using elastic thread or power chain from the arch wire
- If spool elastic is used, it is fed into the bracket, which is without gold chain, manually wound round the arch wire, tied under tension and the excess cut off
- Care must be taken that the 'tied ends' are not sharp and digging into the lips
- The arch wire is checked that it is not too long distally
- All excess wire goes into the sharps box
- *The patient is given oral hygiene instructions and another appointment* (This is usually only a few weeks away as it is important to renew the traction in order to maintain a consistent and sustained 'pull')
- *The patient is shown what has been done and given dietary instructions*

This process is repeated until the tooth has been drawn into the line of the arch.

There is usually a need to reposition the bracket on the exposed canine during the course of this treatment. The subsequent bracket needs to be bonded onto the buccal aspect to achieve full alignment of the tooth.

Buccally positioned canines

If the canine is lying buccally, then it is possible to use a removable appliance prior to a fixed appliance to start extrusion (vertical downward movement) on the upper buccal canine.

If the patient's treatment involves a removable appliance

The nurse needs to prepare:

- *clinical notes*
- *the patient's models*
- *mirror, probe, College tweezers*
- *Adams pliers*

- *spring-forming pliers*
- *Mauns cutters*
- *ruler*
- *dividers*
- *disposable arch wire markers*
- *sharps box*

Chairside procedure

The nurse needs to assist the clinician:

- *Ensure that the patient and clinician are wearing personal protection*
- *Ensure that the patient is seated comfortably in the chair*
- The clinician checks that the wound is clear of debris
- The removable appliance is tried in
- The clasps are adjusted to give maximum retention
- The whip arm is adjusted to fit over the top (gingival) aspect of the bracket
- The end of this is shortened as necessary and cinched, i.e. turned back on itself to avoid a sharp end damaging the soft tissue
- The patient is instructed on how to take the appliance in and out of the mouth
- The patient practices doing this
- They are then shown how to position and place the whip arm
- The whip arm is then activated
- *The patient is given instructions on care of the appliance and oral hygiene*
- *Another appointment is arranged to reactivate the whip arm in a few weeks, in order to maintain continuous force on the tooth*

The widespread popularity of fixed appliance therapy makes it:

- the favoured method to use when drawing ectopic palatal and buccal canines into their correct positions
- essential, if both left and right canines have to be exposed simultaneously and there are other features of a malocclusion that also have to be corrected
- more effective, if they have to be moved heroic distances

ECTOPIC CANINES

Chapter 17
Debonding

When the active phase of fixed appliance treatment is complete, the bonds and bands need to be removed. This process in known as 'debonding'. A long appointment should be scheduled for this much-welcome and long-awaited procedure.

The appointment for the removal of the fixed appliance may be anything from 1 to 2 years after the start of treatment, more if it has been part of a multi-disciplinary treatment. For teenage patients, this represents a significant percentage of their lives. For them, and for the whole team, this appointment is eagerly anticipated!

Occasionally, one dental arch is braced before the other, e.g. if the bite needs to be opened. However, it is uncommon for the two arches to be debonded on separate occasions and as a general rule both upper and lower appliances are removed at the same appointment.

Just as the fitting of the fixed appliance takes longer than the average appointment, so the removal of the appliance needs more time.

The nurse will need to prepare (Figures 17.1 and 17.7):

- *the patient's clinical notes*
- *the patient's model box*
- *mouth mirror, probe and College tweezers*
- *anterior bracket removing pliers (Figure 17.2)*
- *anterior ceramic bracket removing pliers, if needed*
- *band-removing pliers (Figure 17.3)*
- *band-slitting pliers (Figure 17.4)*
- *Mitchell trimmer*
- *adhesive-removing pliers (Figure 17.5)*
- *contra-angled (CA) handpiece and debonding bur (Figure 17.6)*
- *prophylactic paste and rubber cup*
- *sharps container for wire, brackets, etc.*
- *3-in-1 syringe*
- *suction*
- *floss*
- *hand mirror*

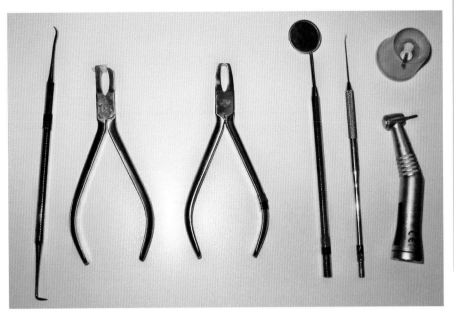

Figure 17.1 Tray for deband.

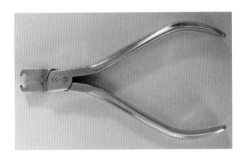

Figure 17.2 Anterior bracket removing pliers.

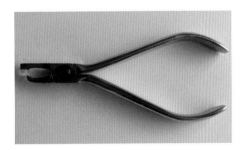

Figure 17.3 Band-removing pliers.

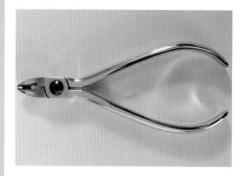

Figure 17.4 Band-slitting pliers.

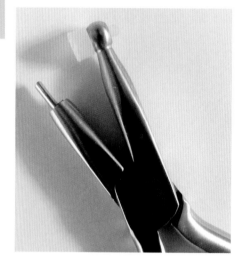

Figure 17.5 Adhesive-removing pliers.

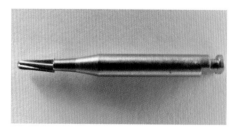

Figure 17.6 Debonding bur.

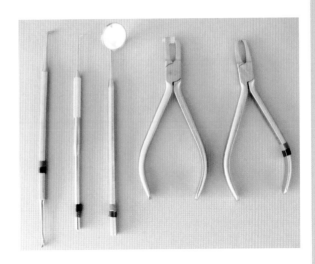

Figure 17.7 Band and bracket removal tray.

- *alginate, bowl and spatula*
- *upper and lower impression trays*
- *wax knife and wax for bite*
- *method of softening wax, blow torch, hot water, etc.*
- *impression disinfectant solution, plastic bag for impressions in transit*
- *laboratory form (to go with impressions to the technician)*
- *camera and lip retractors (if photographic records are needed)*
- *X-ray request form (if end of treatment radiographs are needed at this appointment)*

Procedure

- *Ensure that dentist, nurse and patient are wearing personal protection (it is vital that protective tinted glasses are worn for this procedure)*
- *Make the patient comfortable in the chair*
- Bands are then loosened and subsequently removed from molar teeth along with any residual cement
- Some clinicians remove O-rings or ligatures from around the metal brackets
- Arch wire is removed and then brackets are removed
- Some clinicians remove metal brackets and arch wire together
- Arch wire is often removed from brackets prior to removal of ceramic brackets (non-metal brackets, e.g. ceramic are often more difficult to remove and can 'shatter' in the process. It is vital that adequate eye protection is worn for this procedure)
- Any remaining adherent cement is removed from the molars, using a Mitchell trimmer
- If buccal tubes have been used instead of bands, they are removed
- Any residual adhesive left after the buccal tubes or brackets have been taken off is removed (This is removed by using a slow CA handpiece and

a debonding bur which removes adhesive but does not damage the enamel. Burs can be fine, coarse, rose head or tapered)
- Floss is used between contact points
- Thorough polishing is given, using a CA handpiece, rubber cup and prophylactic paste
- Upper and lower alginate impressions and wax squash bite are then taken
- Impressions and bite are disinfected before going to the laboratory
- *Laboratory form is filled in requesting:*
  - *study models*
  - *upper retainer (Hawley or Essix) (including the design for a Hawley (Figure 17.8))*
  - *lower retainer (usually Essix (Figure 17.9))*
  - *sometimes, a fixed retainer (Figure 17.10)*

Also, the pre- and post-treatment study models have to be filed in the patients model box for quality control and clinical audit. They are then peer assessment rating (PAR) scored to measure how much improvement has been achieved by the orthodontic treatment.

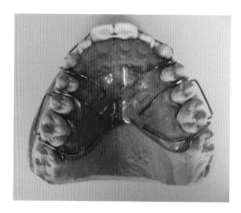

Figure 17.8 Hawley retainer.

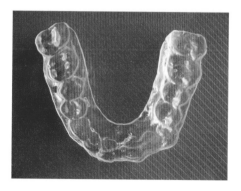

Figure 17.9 Essix retainer.

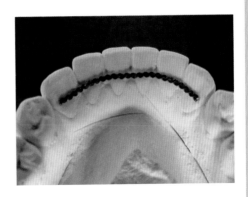

Figure 17.10 Fixed retainer.

A custom-made gum shield can now be organised if the patient plays contact sports. In fixed appliances, an easily mouldable one has been used as the position of the teeth changes so frequently.

If previous photographic records have been taken, post-deband shots can be taken, both intra- and extra-orally.

End of treatment radiographs may be taken at this appointment.

After all traces of the appliance have been removed and the patient has had an opportunity to admire their teeth, there is a further discussion regarding oral hygiene.

For patients who have had the fixed appliances in place for 18 months to 2 years there may be a certain amount of staining on the teeth.

This may be due to:

- black tea
- coffee
- red wine
- curries
- some tomato-based products, such as ketchup
- all foods that have a high level of colouring
- smoking – some patients may have taken it up since their brace was fitted

After the deband appointment, it is important that the teeth are professionally cleaned and polished, and the hygienist removes any calculus that is present on the teeth. Calculus is formed from plaque (a mixture of food, saliva and bacteria) which has been allowed to collect and form around the gingival margin.

It irritates gums and makes them puffy and bleed.

Before fitting the fixed appliances the teeth are cleaned with prophylactic paste that is oil-free. Now, paste that is slightly more abrasive is used.

After the appliance has been removed, patients are encouraged to spend some time flossing their teeth and paying special attention to their gums, before their next appointment when their retainers are fitted and they begin the retention stage of their treatment.

Chapter 18

Retention and retainers

Retention comes after the active treatment is completed, when the appliance is removed.

It is a passive stage and an important part of treatment.

It is crucial because it prevents the teeth from relapsing (moving out of their new position) and returning to the original one.

After the end of active treatment and after debanding, the surrounding tissues have yet to consolidate.

Because teeth have been moved away from their original position, new alveolar bone has to form and consolidate, and the gingival fibres have to adapt.

The teeth need many months to 'firm up', so it is especially important to faithfully wear retainers in the early stages.

The patient must understand that they need to wear the retainers to maintain good results or else everyone's hard work and effort will be undone.

What type of retention and for how long it is to be used is prescribed by the clinician and is part of the treatment plan.

If the patient does not comply with the instructions and the teeth move some way out of alignment, going back into fixed appliances again is often the only way of retrieving the situation. However, the patient may have run out of compliance or, in the National Health Service (NHS)-funded service, the Index of Orthodontic Treatment Need (IOTN) for this would now be scored too low to qualify for treatment.

However, there can be other reasons for results to relapse.

- There can be unfavourable growth, often in the mandible
- Teeth do not fully intercuspate or interdigitate (fit together) in occlusion, so that there is scope for them to slip out of position

There are two terms used to describe how the teeth 'fit' together.
They are:

- intercuspate
- interdigitate

although intercuspate is the correct and preferred term.

When the teeth are in occlusion, they 'mesh', like closing your hands together and putting your fingers between one another (hence, the term interdigitate).

Retainers can be:

- a removable type
- fixed to the teeth

There are no standard criteria set for the length of time you need to wear a retainer.

A longer retention period may be needed depending on the complexity of movement achieved.

For removable retainers, some clinicians say:

- full-time for a year
- then 6 months, nights only
- then discontinue

Others say, full-time for a year, then nights only for 6 months, then reduce the wear down to a couple of nights a week.

Some say that the frequency and time for which retainers are worn can be reduced but never discontinued. It may be only for a couple of nights a week but this is still vital. If for any reason the retainers should suddenly feel tight, then wear them more regularly for a little while until the tightness stops.

This means wearing retainers indefinitely on this occasional basis, may be for life.

It is important to fit the retainers as soon as possible after active treatment has finished and the fixed appliances have been removed.

REMOVABLE RETAINERS

The most common forms are:

- Hawley retainer (Figure 18.1)

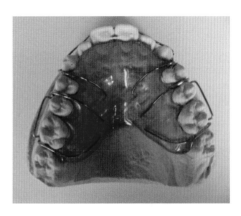

Figure 18.1 Hawley retainer.

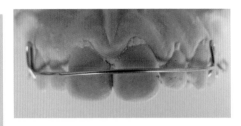

Figure 18.2 Labial bow.

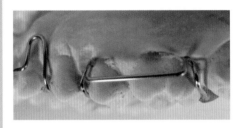

Figure 18.3 Adams crib.

- Essix retainers
- occasionally, removable appliances that have been made passive

HAWLEY RETAINERS

Consist of:

- an acrylic base plate, which fits around the palatal upper and lingual lower gum margins for stability, and incorporates the metal components
- a labial bow which fits over the front of the anterior teeth (Figure 18.2)
- Adams crib, usually positioned on the first molars for retention of the appliance, i.e. keeping it in place (Figure 18.3)

BEGG RETAINERS

Consist of:

- an acrylic baseplate
- a labial bow from the upper second molars with U loops at the first molar regions
- no Adams cribs

These are both:

- worn full-time
- worn when eating
- removed for cleaning
- removed and replaced by a gum shield for contact sports
- quite discreet, as only a thin wire is visible

ESSIX RETAINERS

An Essix retainer:

- is a light, clear 'aligner' type appliance
- does not have any wires
- is a vacuum-formed appliance made from thermo-plastic material

These are:

- lighter
- less visible
- not worn for eating and drinking
- often worn just at night

Essix retainers (Figure 18.4) are sometimes used in the lower arch if:

- it might be hard to get good retention using a Hawley retainer
- the patient would tolerate it better
- an adult patient would find it socially more acceptable

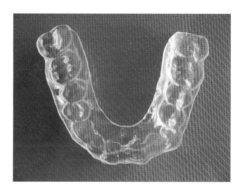

Figure 18.4 Essix retainer.

POSITIONERS

Positioners are sometimes fitted at the end if treatment.

- These are flexible splints which are mildly active
- They continue to correct any small or mild irregularity which still remains after the active appliances have been removed

These devices are made by the technician to a very exact prescription.

MAKING REMOVABLE RETAINERS

For making a removable Hawley or Essix retainer at deband, in addition to the debanding instruments, the nurse will need to prepare:

- *upper and lower impressions*
- *a wax bite*
- *wax knife and method of softening the wax*
- *disinfectant solution for the impressions and bite*
- *a laboratory instruction sheet*

At the fitting of a removable Hawley or Essix retainer, *the nurse needs to prepare:*

- *the patient's clinical notes*
- *the patient's model box*
- *the retainer/retainers from the laboratory*
- *mirror, probe and College tweezers*
- *a protective retainer case for the patient to use when the retainer is not being worn, e.g. while playing contact sports*
- *instruction leaflet*
- *a hand mirror*

plus for a Hawley retainer:

- *Adams pliers (Figure 18.5)*
- *spring-forming pliers*
- *straight handpiece and acrylic bur for adjustments to the acrylic*

Procedure

- *Ensure that the dentist, nurse and patient are wearing personal protective equipment*
- *Esure that the patient is comfortable*
- The retainer is fitted in the mouth
- A check is made that it fits well and is comfortable

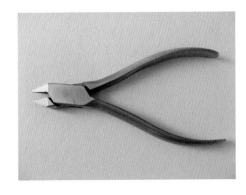

Figure 18.5 Adams plier.

- Any adjustment is then made
- The patient is shown how to remove it (it is always easier at their first attempt for the patient to remove it)
- The patient is shown how to insert it
- *Instruction is given on when to wear it, how to clean it and oral hygiene*
- *An instruction leaflet is also given*
- *The patient is given a protective case*
- *The Medical Devices form is filed in the patient's notes*

For safety, the retainers need to be kept in a firm container when not being worn (Figure 18.6).

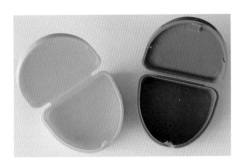

Figure 18.6 Retainer cases.

FIXED RETAINERS

Fixed retainers consist of a fine multi-flex wire or similar flexible length of metal attachment, which is bonded directly onto the lingual or palatal surface of the anterior teeth and which keeps them in position and joined together. They can be used in addition to Essix retainers which are fitted over the fixed retainer.

This is often used when:

- extra retention is needed
- there is a possibility that midline spacing (diastemas) may open (Figure 18.7)

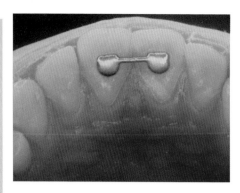

Figure 18.7 Fixed retainer to prevent diastema reopening.

- there has been correction of severely rotated teeth
- the patient may not respond well to wearing a removable retainer adequately
- the occlusal intercuspation may contribute to instability

The fixed retainer (Figures 18.7 and 18.8):

- is not visible, placed on the lingual or palatal surfaces of the teeth
- is small and discreet
- does not interfere with speech
- is not uncomfortable to the tongue
- gives patients peace of mind

However:

- it does need to be regularly checked by the clinicians
- because it is harder to use floss where there is a permanent wire, special efforts must be made with oral hygiene in those areas
- because the adhesives used are similar to those used for a fixed appliance, patients have to avoid the same foods and drinks that may be harmful, e.g. hard, sticky, crunchy or acidic

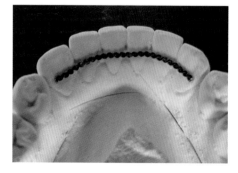

Figure 18.8 Fixed retainer.

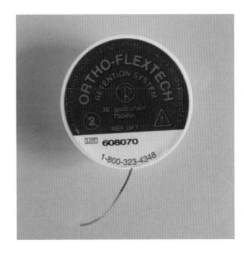

Figure 18.9 Wire for fixed retainers.

Fitting a fixed (bonded) retainer

The fixed retainer is normally fitted at the Deband appointment.

- There are wires commercially available that can be used from the spool and fixed into place (Figure 18.9)
- Some wire-fixed retainers are to be made in the laboratory by the technician; for this an alginate impression for a work model is taken on the last adjustment appointment. The technician fabricates the wire on this model

Multi-strand wire gives flexibility for this, as does flexible, gold-link chain. The fixed palatal retainer must not interfere with the bite of the teeth on closing.

The nurse will need to prepare:

- *the patient's models*
- *the model and retainer from the laboratory, if relevant*
- *the wire for the retainer that the clinician requests or prefers*
- *a 3-in-1 syringe*
- *aspirator*
- *saliva ejectors*
- *cheek retractors*
- *cotton wool rolls*
- *prophylaxis handpiece, rubber cup and paste*
- *hand scaling instruments*
- *CA handpiece, composite finishing burs*
- *disposable Dappen's pots*
- *etchant and primer or self etch primer*
- *adhesive – there are ones specifically for lingual retainers*

- *mirror, probe and College tweezers*
- *floss*
- *light-emitting diode (LED) light*
- *special protective glasses for clinician, patient and nurse*
- *Weingart pliers*
- *light-wire cutters*
- *light-wire pliers*
- *flat plastic*

Procedure

- *Ensure the dentist, nurse and patient wear personal protective equipment*
- *Make the patient comfortable*
- After the upper and lower fixed appliances have been removed, the teeth are cleaned using rubber cup and prophylaxis paste after using scalers (mostly in adult patients) to remove any deposits of calculus
- Cheek retractors, saliva ejectors, cotton rolls, etc., are put in to maintain a dry field
- The wire previously made on the model is tried in or wire or gold chain is then cut and customised to fit exactly and is tried in
- The area is etched, washed and re-dried
- The area is primed or self-etch primer applied
- Adhesive is applied to lingual of each tooth to be included in the bonding process

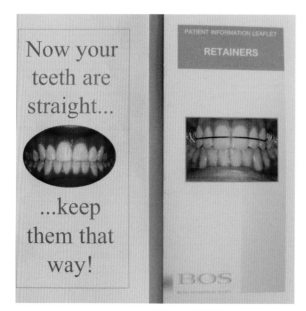

Figure 18.10 Retainer leaflets. (Reproduced with the kind permission of Ortho-Care and of the British Orthodontic Society.)

- The wire is seated into the adhesive on the teeth
- Some clinicians use interproximal floss to stabilise the wire
- Adhesive is cured with LED light
- Any further adhesive that is required is added
- The added adhesive is cured
- The retainer is checked to ensure it is not rough to the tongue and soft tissues
- If the patient is to also have an Essix retainer:
  - upper and lower alginate impressions are taken
  - wax bite is taken to record the occlusion
- *The patient is given instructions on how to maintain the retainer*
- *The patient is given the leaflet (Figure 18.10) and an appointment to check the fixed retainer in the future*

Chapter 19

Aligners

In addition to the conventional systems of removable and fixed appliances, there are now methods of straightening and de-rotating overcrowded teeth by using aligners.

Most aligners are similar in appearance to Essix retainers and are made of flexible plastic. There are some aligners that are made from acrylic.

They are both removable.

They are usually used as a non-extraction treatment option for patients with:

- mild spacing
- mild crowding
- mild rotations

They do not aim to treat patients with severe crowding or skeletal discrepancy.

Aligners are popular with adults because:

- they are less visible
- they can be taken out for special occasions, e.g. meetings, dates
- they are easy to use and don't affect speech
- apart from when eating and drinking, they can be worn all the time

Advantages

The advantages of this system are:

- surgery time, both for the patient and the clinician, can be saved on adjustment appointments
- the aligners are comfortable, with no sharp wires or brackets to cause discomfort
- aesthetically, they are very discreet
- easy to keep clean

Disadvantages

The disadvantages of this system are:

- should an aligner not be worn sufficiently, it cannot produce enough force to achieve steady progress

- if an aligner is accidentally lost, another one has to be ordered and made, which takes time and incurs an additional cost
- there is no control over tooth root movements (as there is with fixed appliance therapy)
- it is limited in the degree of movements it can achieve

TYPES OF ALIGNERS

Type one

The first type, known under trade names such as:

- Invisalign
- ClearStep

use a series of appliances.

Teeth can be aligned using a series of aligners that move them small amounts at a time.

How far the teeth are crowded and rotated would govern how many aligners are needed.

When the first one is fitted, it can feel a little tight and there is significant pressure on the teeth.

After a few days, this becomes less as the teeth are moving towards their new position.

After a fortnight or so, the next aligner is fitted; again, it feels tight and this gets less as the teeth move.

This goes on until the teeth are in their new alignment and are straight.

Type two

The second type, like the one marketed under the name, the Inman Aligner, uses just one appliance.

The Inman Aligner is also a removable appliance. It must be worn as much as possible.

It has a bar over the front of the teeth and uses the force produced by a coiled spring to push and pull the teeth and compress them into alignment.

This method is most successful when aligning the anterior segments.

The patient must visit the surgery regularly to check the aligner's progress.

The scope and therefore the length of treatment are shorter than other methods.

For both methods, there are small firm foam cylinders available. The patient chews on these and the action of this is said to help seat the aligners.

INTERPROXIMAL STRIPPING OR INTERDENTAL ENAMEL REDUCTION

For both methods, in order to move crowded teeth into a better position, there is a need create some space.

The method of getting this small amount of space is known as interproximal stripping or interdental enamel reduction.

This needs to be done, to a greater or lesser degree depending on the space needed. As the aligners move the teeth, they gradually use up the extra space created.

This technique can also be used selectively in fixed appliance therapy if there is:

- an area of very mild, localised crowding
- the need to de-rotate an individual tooth

Sometimes, in order to eliminate 'dark triangles' gingivally, contact points are reduced so that the teeth can come closer together and provide an improved shape of the papilla. Interdental enamel reduction can also be employed when re-shaping and contouring.

Stripping or slenderising removes tiny amounts of proximal enamel from:

- either the mesial or distal contact point, or both, of the tooth
- the adjacent tooth, if more appropriate

This can be done either:

- contra-angled handpiece
- using an air rotor
  or
- manually

The handpiece method is becoming more widespread as:

- it is easier to use at the back of the mouth
- the oscillating movement causes less striation of the enamel
- it is less likely to cause periodontal damage

AIR ROTOR

- contra-angled handpiece
- cutting discs
- contouring discs

- fine tapered diamond burs
- finishing burs

are used.

When discs are used, a guard must be in place to protect the patients' soft tissues.

Up to 8 mm, spread amongst several teeth, can be gained in an arch.

This technique does not cause such striations on the enamel surface as the manual method.

MANUAL

This method is slower and may be easier when monitoring the amount of enamel to be removed.

The interproximal strips:

- are made of stainless steel, usually diamond-coated
- some are single use
- some can be autoclaved
- are of varying thickness
- come in a fine or coarse texture
- are either single or double sided
- can be saw strips
- sometimes, serrated strips

They can be used as long strips:

- where the clinician holds each end and uses a 'sawing' action
- where the blade is inserted into a hand-held instrument

There is:

- an anterior instrument
- a posterior instrument

The posterior instrument has to work on teeth at the back of the mouth where access may be difficult, so it is angled to give greater ease of working.

There are several instruments available which are designed to accurately measure the amount of space that needs to be achieved pre- and post-stripping. These include:

- an incremental thickness gauge
  - This is a set of graded stainless steel gauges, like small rulers, that fit in between the teeth after stripping, to measure the gap

ALIGNERS

- an interdental measurement instrument
  - This is a hand-held instrument with a conical end. The amount it can be inserted in the gap between the teeth calculates the space achieved

After this treatment, patients are advised to use gel to assist with remineralisation of the enamel.

This gel is similar to that used by patients:

- with decalcification
- who have had a course of tooth whitening

The gel is easily applied using a manual toothbrush.

START OF TREATMENT

After the initial assessment of the teeth and a treatment plan has been made, the patient needs to have records taken.

TYPE ONE

If they are having a series of aligners, *the nurse needs to prepare:*

- *alginate, bowls and spatula (putty may be preferred)*
- *upper and lower impression trays*
- *a wax squash bite*
- *wax knife and method of softening wax*
- *solution to disinfectant impressions and bite*
- *plastic bag and laboratory work sheet*
- *have the radiographs available*
- *camera*
- *cheek retractors*
- *mouth mirror*

The impression and bite registrations are all sent to the laboratory along with a detailed treatment and instruction plan.

The technicians will then, using computer software:

- create a model of the desired finished result
- calculate the required movement each aligner must be programmed to make to achieve this
- calculate the number of aligners that will be needed
- calculate how much interproximal stripping is needed (if it is needed)

This is done until the measurements, for a series of aligners that will move the teeth into the positions of the required finished result, on the generated model, are complete. The calculations are then transferred to their laboratory where the aligners are manufactured. This work is sometimes sent to a specialist laboratory overseas.

In this way, a series of aligners is made.

These are:

- bespoke
- graded
- to be used in sequence
- all made at the same time
- sent back to the clinician

Each aligner will move the teeth an exact amount. Before the aligner is fitted, the interproximal adjustment (if needed) has to be made, precisely as prescribed. The teeth are then moved into this space.

The patient then returns to the surgery at regular intervals to check and monitor progress.

When the aligner has achieved its tooth movement, the clinician may again make an exact interproximal adjustment and then go onto the next aligner in the series.

Like all orthodontic treatment, once the teeth are in the right place, there must be a period of retention to prevent them relapsing and slipping out of position again.

TYPE TWO

The Single Appliance Aligner, e.g. the Inman Aligner

Sometimes, patients have a single aligner, rather than a series of aligners, e.g. an Inman Aligner, which is made in the laboratory and has acrylic and wire components.

Unlike the multi aligner system, this one relies on the following:

- the aligner has movable parts
- it uses piston like NiTi coil springs
- it has labial and lingual components
- all movements are being achieved with the single appliance

It consists of a baseplate and moving parts. The lingual coil spring puts controlled pressure on the lingual aspects of teeth while a labial bar exerts pressure that pushes against this. In this way, the teeth become 'squeezed' between the two, so are eased into alignment.

To begin this treatment, *the nurse needs to prepare:*

- *the patient's model box*
- *upper and lower impression trays*
- *alginate, bowl and spatula (putty if preferred)*
- *wax for bite recording*
- *disinfectant solution for impressions and bite*
- *bag and laboratory instructions*
- *form for instructions for the technician*

Chairside procedure

- *The nurse needs to:*
- *ensure that the dentist, patient and nurse have personal protective equipment*
- *make sure that the patient is sitting comfortably*
- Upper and lower impressions for study and work models are taken
- Bite registration is recorded
- *The impressions and bite are disinfected and bagged*
- *Ensure that the laboratory sheet is filled in*
- Intra- and extra-oral photographs are taken
- *The patient is given instructions on the new appliance and told what to expect at the next visit*
- *The next appointment is confirmed*

The impressions then go to the technician. When the patient returns for the fitting appointment

the nurse needs to prepare:

- *the aligner to be fitted*
- *the patient's model box*
- *mouth mirror*
- *ruler*
- *Adams pliers*
- *stripping kit, if required*
- *oscillating handpiece and shaped burs*
- *handpiece and acrylic bur*
- *hand mirror*
- *patient instruction leaflets*

Procedure

- *Ensure that the dentist, patient, and nurse have personal protective equipment*
- *Make sure that the patient is sitting comfortably*

- *Have the work from the laboratory*
- Use stripping kit or oscillating handpiece as required
- Fit the Aligner
- Trim with acrylic bur if necessary
- Use Adams pliers to adjust the appliance as necessary
- Use ruler to record spaces and rotations
- *Give the patient instructions on how to remove and insert the appliances*
- *Give instruction leaflet on how to clean and care for the appliances, plus leaflet*
- *Book the next appointment*

The patient must be seen at regular intervals.

When the required alignment has been achieved, the patient must have impressions taken for:

- retainers
- end-of-treatment study models

As with all appliances and aligners made in a laboratory, they must have a Medical Devices certificate issued when they are made.

These record:

- the materials used and their properties
- their batch numbers
- who made the appliances

These must always be filed in the patients, notes after fitting the appliance.

ALIGNERS

Chapter 20
Multi-disciplinary orthodontics

Orthodontic treatment is often part of a multi-disciplinary team approach for dental patients.

These patients fall into three main categories of combined need:

- Restorative
- Surgical
- Cleft

Some patients, for example patients with a cleft condition, may require treatment from all three categories.

RESTORATIVE

Some simple cases are multi-disciplinary between the general dental practitioner (GDP) and the orthodontist but more severe cases are seen at an orthodontic/restorative multi-disciplinary clinic for full assessment.

Microdontia

These patients sometimes have conical or 'spiky' teeth. The most common tooth affected is the upper lateral incisor. These teeth are sometimes referred to as peg-shaped. These irregularly shaped teeth have to be built up either with facings, veneers or crowns. Sometimes, several teeth are affected.

Hypodontia

These patients do not have all the teeth needed to make up the full dentition. They rarely have both the deciduous (baby) and permanent tooth missing. If this is just a single tooth, it may be possible to close the space orthodontically. If the span is too wide, then it is necessary to have some type of replacement.

This could be:

- a denture
- a bridge
- an implant

Some patients with hypodontia have several missing teeth, even three or more per quadrant. Sometimes, hypodontia and microdontia are found in the same patient. Orthodontic treatment can be invaluable in correcting the existing permanent teeth into position to facilitate the restoration of spaces left by the absence of a number of teeth.

SURGICAL

Some patients are born with:

- a facial deformity
- skeletal pattern imbalance
- problems with condyles
- unfavourable growth (especially in the mandible)

These may require corrective jaw surgery.

It may also be necessary to have surgery on:

- ectopic teeth which need surgical uncovering and exposure
- teeth which need transplanting to a more favourable position
- a thick, fleshy frenum
- supernumerary, submerged or impacted teeth

A frequent interface between the orthodontist and the maxillo-facial surgical team comes when the patient requires an osteotomy. This is a procedure to correct a skeletal discrepancy of mandible/maxilla. Patients are seen on a combined clinic. At these clinics, the patients are also given information leaflets (Figure 20.1).

Most osteotomies are carried out inside the mouth. Sometimes, bone is harvested from another site, often from the hip (the iliac crest) for use in the procedure.

These are carried out after the patient has finished most of their growth. In the case of the face, this is later for boys than girls.

They can be:

- maxillary
- mandibular
- both (known as bimaxillary)

MULTI-DISCIPLINARY ORTHODONTICS

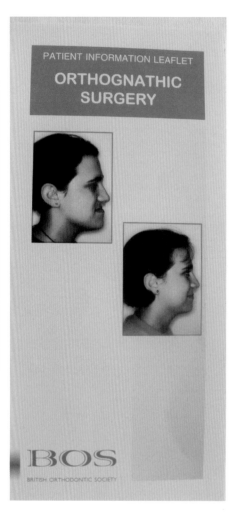

Figure 20.1 Leaflet for orthognathic surgery. (Reproduced with the kind permission of the British Orthodontic Society.)

The maxillary (midface) osteotomies include:

- Le Fort I (involving the tooth-bearing maxilla)
- Le Fort II (involving the maxilla and the nose)
- Le Fort III (involving the maxilla, nose and cheeks)

The mandibular (lower face) osteotomies include:

- sagittal split (centred at the angles and ascending ramus of the mandible)
- genioplasty (when the tip of the chin is repositioned)

For many patients, these operations will alter their appearance. This is one of the reasons the patient may be offered an appointment with a clinical psychologist at this stage.

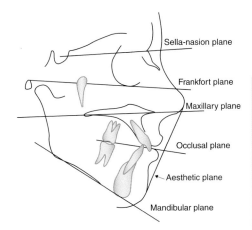

Sella-nasion plane

Frankfort plane

Maxillary plane

Occlusal plane

Aesthetic plane

Mandibular plane

Figure 20.2 Drawing showing Frankfort plane.

MULTI-DISCIPLINARY ORTHODONTICS

For these patients, the orthodontist and maxillo-facial surgeon need to see patients together to formulate a treatment plan.

As part of this, the orthodontist will take radiographs, including a lateral and, occasionally, a postero-anterior (PA) cephalogram on which to reproduce a tracing.

There are many reference points on a tracing.

Skeletal measurements can be recorded:

- horizontally, vertically, antero-posterior (front to back)
- transverse, across width (less commonly used)

For the purposes of a basic guide, it would be useful as a baseline to see the:

- Frankfort plane (Figure 20.2) – as the horizontal measurement
- maxillary plane – as a line from the posterior border to the anteriorpoint of the hard palate
- occlusal plane – as a line between the teeth in occlusion
- mandibular plane – as the lower border of the mandible
- aesthetic plane – as a line along the soft tissue profile from the tip of the nose to the tip of the chin

Tracing can be done either:

- manually

or

- using computer software

In order to make a manual tracing, the operator will need:

- tracing film (usually 8 × 10″)
- a tooth-tracing template
- triangle

- cephalometric protractor and template (joined)
- metric scale rule
- yellow graph pencil
- a light box

When using the manual method the clinician will:

- manually place the lateral cephalometric (side view of the head) radiograph on the light box (with the nose facing to the right)
- place the tracing paper over this
- then using a series of recognised hard tissue coordinate points, trace lines between these points and measure the relevant angles
- using a tooth template, protractor and pencil, then produce a tracing which will accurately show the pre-surgical measurements of the patient and this helps form the proposed orthodontic and surgical planning

NB: Soft tissue profiles are not so predictable but as a guide, follow the bone changes by 50%.

When using a computer, the operator needs to trace the reference points which are plotted by the software program. This calculates the angles and measurements, which, when printed out are shown together with line tracings.

In addition, the laboratory technician:

- may also be asked to make a Kesling set-up
- This is done by taking a set of work models, cutting off and 'resetting' the teeth in their projected position

Orthodontic treatment will then be planned and carried out by putting the teeth in the positions they need to be in prior to the surgery.

The aim of the procedure is to align the dental arches so they are coordinated and fit together at operation. This makes the post-surgical orthodontic stage simpler and shorter.

PRE-SURGICAL ORTHODONTICS

For the nurse, these appointments need the same preparation as for a routine fixed appliance.

When the orthodontist is satisfied that the teeth are in the planned position prior to surgery, they then take impressions.

COORDINATION IMPRESSIONS

Coordination impressions are:

- usually taken with the arch wires in the mouth
- are of upper and lower alginate
- have a wax squash bite

These are:

- cast by the technician
- the coordination models are checked by the orthodontist to ensure that the positioning of the teeth is correct and the proposed occlusion is correct for the planned surgical procedure

If this is so, then an operation date is arranged with the surgeon after they have reviewed the patient at this stage.

Coordination and communication is essential.

All appointments between the two specialties, the laboratory and the patient, have to be coordinated.

COUNTDOWN TO SURGERY

With:

- the pre-surgical orthodontics completed and
- an appointment date booked for surgery

an appointment is made for further impressions a few weeks before the operation date. These are known as wafer impressions.

For this appointment, the nurse needs to prepare:

- *the patient's model box*
- *a fixed appliance tray*
- *mirror, probe, College tweezers*
- *distal-end pliers*
- *light-wire pliers*
- *Weingart pliers*
- *ligatures*
- *Kobyashi ligatures*
- *Mathieu/mosquito/haemostat*
- *ligature director*
- *alginate, bowls and spatula*
- *upper and lower impression trays*

- *wax for bite registration*
- *solution to disinfect the impressions and bite*
- *equipment for taking face bow reading if necessary*
- *sharps box*
- *clinical camera*
- *photographic mirrors*
- *lip retractors*
- *patient relief wax*

Chairside procedure

- The arch wires are removed from both the maxilla and the mandible
- Upper and lower alginate impressions are taken for the wafer, the planning models and orthodontic study models
- A bite registration is taken
- The arch wires are then 'tied in' (for strength, metal ligatures, often with Kobyashi hooks, are used to hold the arch wires securely in the brackets)
- Alternatively, crimpable hooks will be added to the arch wire instead of using Kobyashi hooks (it is important that the appliance is robust and remains intact for the surgical operation and post-surgical orthodontic stage)
- Intra- and extra-oral photographs are then taken

NB: If the patient is having a bimaxillary procedure, then a face bow measurement will also be taken.

The patient has now completed the pre-surgical phase of orthodontic treatment and is ready for the operation.

The impressions and bite then go to the laboratory where an acrylic wafer is made and model planning carried out in conjunction with the surgeon and orthodontist. This is to determine the correct occlusal position to set the jaw during operation.

This wafer will be used by the surgeon during the surgery. It is made of clear plastic.

It is placed between the teeth and used in theatre as a location 'guide' for the occlusion.

Try-in of wafer

A week before the scheduled operation date, the wafer is 'tried in' to make sure that it fits correctly.

THE OPERATION

- Most osteotomies are approached from inside the mouth
- Patients do sometimes have external drains
- The bony sections are normally plated (rigid fixation)
- Afterwards, the patients will also be in intermaxillary elastics where the upper and lower dental arches will be held together immediately post surgery
- These will be removed when the sutures are removed and then replaced by new ones, under the guidance of the orthodontist
- How long the patient wears these depends on a number of factors, such as how quickly they are healing, how extensive the operation and how much post-operation orthodontic movement may be needed

POST-OP APPOINTMENT

About 10 days after the operation, the patient has an appointment with the orthodontist.

The nurse needs to prepare:

- *the patient's clinical notes*
- *radiographs*
- *the orthodontic planning model box*
- *the surgical planning box*
- *a fixed appliance tray*
- *intermaxillary elastics*
- *hand mirror*
- *clinical camera*
- *photographic cheek retractors*
- *photographic mirrors*

Chairside procedure

- *The dentist, nurse and patient wear personal protective equipment*
- *The patient is made comfortable in the chair*
- The occlusion is checked (the patient may still be swollen and sore)
- The clinician may wish to alter or reposition the elastics pattern
- Cheeks and lips are checked for normal sensation (sometimes, they have 'numb' or 'tingling' areas post op)
- Advice on oral hygiene and diet is given (appropriate radiographs have usually been taken by the surgical team)
- The patient may have photographs taken

MULTI-DISCIPLINARY ORTHODONTICS

A further follow-up appointment is arranged with the patient.

The patient will continue to be bruised and to feel swollen for some time how much and for how long varies from patient to patient. This will eventually subside. However, the loss of feeling around the face, especially the lips and chin, may take longer to return to normal. Some patients notice tingling and feeling slowly returning up to a year after surgery. Care must be taken not to bite or burn their lips when eating and drinking.

The patient will have been given dietary and oral hygiene advice. In time, they will also be given instruction and will be able to change their own elastics for the time that they are needed.

POST-SURGICAL ORTHODONTICS

- Usually, there is a period of post-surgical orthodontics to 'sock in' the bite and make sure that the bite fully intercuspates
- This can be anything from 3–8 months
- The patient is then ready for debanding of the fixed appliances and the fitting of retention appliances

There is a protocol as to when the patients are seen on combined clinics, where they are monitored and reviewed by the whole multi-disciplinary team. The final review appointment is normally 2 years after debonding and further advice on retainer wear is given before discharge.

OTHER SURGICAL PROCEDURES UNDERTAKEN IN THEATRE

Sometimes, patients have to have surgical extraction of:

- severely submerged teeth
- impacted teeth and buried supernumerary teeth

The following may be undertaken under general anaesthesia in theatre or, under local anaesthesia.

- Frenectomy (removal of frenum which can be implicated in a diastema or preventing space closure)
- Removal of tongue tie (if this is causing serious clinical difficulties)

UNCOVERING ECTOPIC CANINES

Patients can also have surgical uncovering of unerupted ectopic canines (Figure 20.3). When these are exposed, a bracket (which is often attached to a

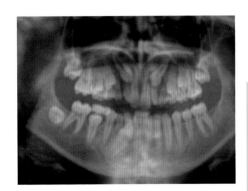

Figure 20.3 Radiograph of ectopic canines.

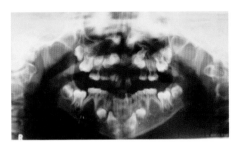

Figure 20.4 Radiograph of patient with cleft.

MULTI-DISCIPLINARY ORTHODONTICS

gold-plated chain), is fitted onto the tooth/teeth. A week or 10 days after surgery, the patient has an orthodontic appointment when traction is applied to the chain from the pre-fitted fixed appliance and the process of drawing the canine into its correct position begins. As the distance shortens, the links of chain are to reduced (see also Chapter 16).

CLEFT LIP AND PALATE

Cleft lip and palate babies are referred to the cleft team as soon as they are born and have a lot of their specialist care undertaken in hospital (Figure 20.4). They will also need routine dental check-ups with a GDP.

The cleft team may consist of:

- a cleft surgeon
- specialist cleft nurses
- an ear, nose and throat (ENT) surgeon
- paediatric audiologist
- an orthodontist
- orthodontic nurses
- a paediatrician
- a paediatric dentist
- feeding advisors

- speech and language therapists (SALT)
- a geneticist

The interface between these specialties provides the care pathway for these patients, which begins at birth and continues until they have completed their treatment, often in the late teens and early twenties.

Some parents are aware that their baby has a cleft before he/she is delivered, because cleft lips can be detected on foetal scans. For others, it is a complete shock. Cleft lip and palate is the most common congenital craniofacial deformity and affects all ethnic groups. Cleft surgeons can come from either maxillo-facial or plastic surgery backgrounds.

There are variations of clefting deformity, which is caused by abnormal facial development before birth. Clefts can also be a symptom of a syndrome or sequence, e.g. Pierre Robin.

The word cleft means a gap or fissure, where there has not been correct fusion between natural structures. This can manifest as:

- a cleft lip – cheiloschisis
- a cleft palate – palatoschisis

Some babies are born with both ranging from:

- a small notch in the upper lip

to

- total bilateral cleft lip and alveolus, and extending to the hard and soft palates

Patients can present with:

- cleft lip (Figure 20.5), unilateral or bilateral
- cleft lip, unilateral or bilateral, plus hard or soft palate (Figures 20.6 and 20.7), or both
- cleft palate only, hard or soft, or both

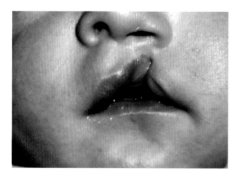

Figure 20.5 Cleft lip.

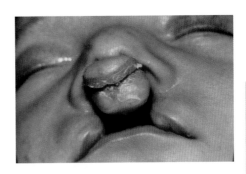

Figure 20.6 Bilateral cleft.

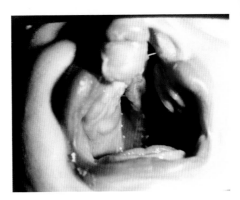

Figure 20.7 Cleft of lip, hard and soft palates.

Clefts can involve:

- the maxillo-facial skeleton
- soft tissue envelope
- the nasal structure
- the hard and soft palates
- the alveolar ridge
- the upper dental arch

This cohort of patients will potentially have a series of operations and procedures over a period lasting from soon after are born until they are in their late teens. They have a lot to cope with apart from their teeth.

Often, they have:

- problems with feeding (as babies). Use Haberman bottles and teats specially designed for them
- problems with speech and being understood
- problems with hearing (glue ear, etc.)
- social difficulties, e.g. teasing
- surgical procedures, bone-harvesting osteotomies, etc.
- problems with plaque control which affects oral hygiene
- hypoplastic, peg-shaped or absent teeth

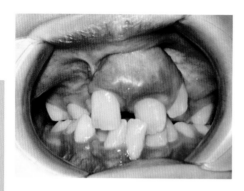

Figure 20.8 Cleft patient prior to orthodontic treatment.

- teeth which may have short or abnormal clinical crowns
- issues surrounding low self-esteem

There is a considerable orthodontic interface with cleft patients to help achieve an aesthetic result which will add to the patients self-esteem (Figure 20.8).

At 9–10 years, they may be treated with orthodontics and bone grafting.

At 15–18 years, they can be treated with orthodontics and osteotomy.

To comply with audit requirements, baseline records are taken for these patients at prescribed intervals.

Problems for the orthodontist:

- lack of alveolar bone at site of cleft means bone grafting is needed
- teeth missing at site of cleft – how to fill the space
  - space closure orthodontically
  - implants
  - acid-etch-retained bridges
- mid-facial growth disrupted due to surgical interventions, e.g. maxillary retrusion
- teeth not in alignment – upper arch narrow and deformed, and tending to crossbites

The nurse needs to prepare the same tray systems for these patients for every stage of appliance treatment as would be needed for routine patients without a cleft.

Cleft patients may need to have additional visits to other specialties as part of their treatment, e.g.:

- speech therapy
- problems with ear and nose

In England and Wales, the CRANE database holds details of adults and children with a cleft lip and/or palate. This is funded by the NHS and is held at the Royal College of Surgeons (England). CLAPA is the representative organisation for all people with and affected by cleft lip and/or palate in the UK.

MULTI-DISCIPLINARY ORTHODONTICS

Chapter 21
Adult orthodontics

Orthodontic treatment is not confined to children and adolescents.

Many adult patients seek an orthodontic solution to improve their function and appearance.

These patients may have discussed their concerns with their dentist (GDP). Often, they may have:

- been denied access to orthodontic treatment as children
- been offered it but they refused to take it up
- had orthodontics with a treatment plan that was incorrect or unsuccessful
- failed to complete treatment or to wear their retainers and the teeth relapsed

Often, patients have been considering an orthodontic treatment option for some time before they actually speak with their dentist.

The dentist will know where it is appropriate to refer the patient, i.e. the severity of the malocclusion.

If it is a relatively mild malocclusion involving:

- mild rotations
- crowding
- spacing

the patient may be referred to a Specialist Practitioner, who has qualified as a dentist and then gone on with post-graduate training in order to achieve a post-graduate qualification in orthodontics.

If it is a more challenging malocclusion involving:

- an underlying skeletal asymmetry
- a complex occlusal problem
- a severe degree of crowding
- a number of congenitally missing teeth
- any untreated ectopic teeth
- signs of bone loss or a periodontal condition

The patient may then be referred to a Consultant Orthodontist, who:

- has qualified as a dentist
- has gone on to achieve further orthodontic qualifications
- has worked in the hospital service as a Senior or Specialist Registrar
- ultimately, be appointed as a Consultant

The treatment plan that they provide will help decide where best to treat the patient.

Adult patients have some advantages over children. They:

- are compliant and keen
- know what they want
- can have interproximal enamel reduction
- have good oral hygiene

They also have some disadvantages. They may have:

- missing teeth
- fractured teeth which are sometimes non-vital
- root-treated teeth
- periodontal disease with resultant gum recession
- implants
- loss of alveolar ridge due to earlier extraction of teeth
- tooth surface loss
- underlying medical health problems
- they have finished facial growth
- teeth which have suffered trauma and have become ankylosed, i.e. fused to the surrounding tissue; these teeth cannot be moved orthodontically
- bridgework; so in some areas, movement and space is compromised
- root resorption and low bone levels
- Temporo-mandibular-joint problems, e.g. pain on opening, clicking, etc.
- para functional habits, e.g. bruxism
- effects on periodontal health if the patient is a smoker

For adult patients, a more socially acceptable and discreet option may include:

- fixed appliances using aesthetic brackets (these can be upper anteriors only) (Figure 21.1)
- bond full upper and lower ceramic brackets (Figure 21.2)

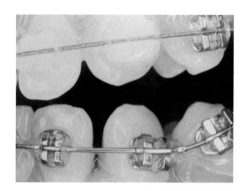

Figure 21.1 Bonding using both metal and aesthetic brackets.

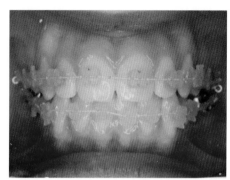

Figure 21.2 Upper and lower aesthetic brackets.

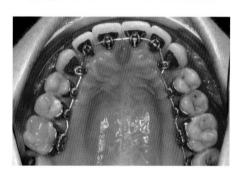

Figure 21.3 Lingual appliance with gold brackets.

ADULT ORTHODONTICS

- removable appliances, i.e. they can be removed for critical business or social meetings
- aligners
- lingual fixed appliances (Figure 21.3)

Adult patients come to seek advice and information for a variety of reasons.

The most common reason is to improve appearance.
Patients may:

- confide that they are embarrassed to smile in public
- want to smile with more confidence

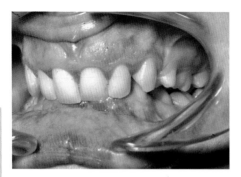

Figure 21.4 Bite stripping labial gingivae.

- have seen a recent photograph of themselves and realise how poor their smile is and how unhappy they are with it
- have a major life event coming, e.g. they are getting married and want to improve their appearance
- not have been offered the access or opportunity to have orthodontic treatment when they were younger
- suffer discomfort from a traumatic occlusion

TO REHABILITATE A TRAUMATIC BITE

Sometimes, the patient bites in a way that is self-damaging. The longer they do it the more damage, often irreversible, is done to teeth, gingivae and palatal soft tissue (Figure 21.4). Patients complain that they suffer more discomfort when they have a cold and the mucosa in the mouth is inflamed.

THE PATIENT MAY BE INVESTIGATING ALL THE OPTIONS

It can be that during the initial consultation with the dentist, the restorative options discussed included provision of crowns, bridges, veneers and implants or a combination of these. Orthodontic treatment may be put forward as an option to achieve an acceptable aesthetic solution and more and more adult patients are exploring this option.

PROBLEMS WITH EATING

Adult patients who have lived with crooked teeth and poor bites for many years may complain that they feel uncomfortable eating in public. As teenagers their

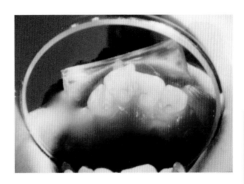

Figure 21.5 Caries between overlapping teeth.

diet would have been less challenging and there were probably fewer social situations which highlighted these difficulties. A common complaint for some patients is that they are unable to 'bite right through a sandwich'; they manage the bread but not always a fibrous filling or lettuce. Sometimes, their malocclusion does not efficiently deal with mastication and food may not have been chewed properly prior to swallowing, which may lead to problems with digestion.

ORAL HYGIENE

Some patients are very aware that their teeth are prone to trapping food after meals. For example, they get fibres of meat or pieces of spinach caught between the teeth during and after meal. This can be socially embarrassing. Flossing between overlapping teeth can be difficult and this may lead to localised periodontal problems. Despite patients' best efforts, rotated and overlapping teeth tend to develop cavities (Figure 21.5) and these are hard for the dentist to fill due to poor access.

WISDOM TEETH

Some patients who have straight teeth worry that the eruption of third molars (wisdom teeth) in their mid-twenties may cause a 'bunching' effect. The National Institute for Health and Clinical Excellence (NICE) has produced guidelines saying that this is not the case, and wisdom teeth are only extracted if they are causing a proven clinical problem.

LOSS OF RETAINED DECIDUOUS TEETH

Some retained deciduous teeth, although severely worn down can last into middle age. Many have no permanent tooth to replace it. However, when they are lost, they cause a problem; what to do with the space they have left? For some patients, the option of closing the space may seem to be preferable to a bridge or an implant. Orthodontics would give them a lasting solution and there would be no need for restorative work, which may have to be replaced over time and also have an ongoing cost implication.

Alternatively, the space may need to be opened further in order to place a satisfactory restoration or implant.

TO ASSIST THE DENTIST IN CARRYING OUT ROUTINE TREATMENT

If a tilted tooth is to be used as an abutment tooth for bridgework, it may need to first be uprighted to allow good parallel preparation of the tooth. Uprighting can be achieved orthodontically. Otherwise, if it is severely tipped there is the possibility that when preparing the tooth the angle might necessitate having to do root canal treatment.

RELAPSED ORTHODONTIC TREATMENT

Some patients have undergone orthodontic treatment as children but there has been relapse and sometimes the original problems may have returned, for what-ever reason. These patients are fairly knowledgeable about what orthodontic treatment entails.

Adults who are considering orthodontic treatment have usually done some research of their own. The internet is a useful source of information and provides them with a basic understanding of what treatment they might expect.

However, adults have different needs and aspirations from children.

They need:

- more discussion and use of demonstration models (Figure 21.6)
- visual presentations
- written leaflets

Sometimes, a friend or colleague will have told them about the treatment they themselves are receiving and this will prompt the patient to think about maybe having something similar for themselves.

So, they may present with a list of 'can I have ...?' questions.

Often, adult patients insist on less visible appliances.

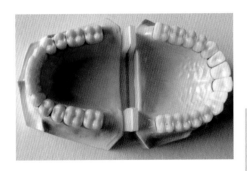

Figure 21.6 Demonstration models.

With adult patients, treatment may appear similar to that of children but their treatment plans are often 'custom made' for them. Some adults may choose to have severely rotated teeth treated but leave a diastema. This would normally be closed in a younger patient but, as this has become part of their accepted appearance it is not seen as needing correction, it is 'part' of them.

Adult patients:

- are self-motivating
- rarely face a problem of oral hygiene, although staining from black coffee and red wine can be a problem!
- can see the benefits and value of having the treatment
- are not going to take risks with diet, oral hygiene or not wearing the appliances as instructed
- are very rewarding patients to treat and they value their smile, albeit arriving a few years later than might have been the case

ADULT ORTHODONTICS

Chapter 22

Mandibular advancement devices

Increasingly, in recent years:

- doctors
- dentists
- respiratory physicians
- ear, nose and throat surgeons

have been seeing patients who are worried that their husband/wife/partner/ friend or relative have disturbed sleep and/or snore.

They are concerned about:

- the noise from snoring which can range from gentle and rhythmic to very loud
- a tendency to 'stop breathing' when asleep, obstructive sleep apnoea (OSA). The patient stops mid snore for a few seconds, snorts or gasps and wake themselves up, and then fall asleep again. This can be repeated several times in an hour

Very often, it is not the patient who complains. They may feel tired but they do not always have broken sleep. It is the person who is kept awake that often gets the snorer to seek advice.

The first step is to see their own doctor (GP) to see what help is available.

These patients are then referred to a Sleep Clinic, usually at their local hospital and there they are assessed by a physician and a specialist sleep nurse.

They fill in an Epworth Sleepiness Test.

Patients use the following scale to choose the most appropriate number to assess how they react in certain situations. These range from:

- 0 – would never doze or sleep
- 1 – slight chance of dozing or sleeping
- 2 – moderate chance of dozing or sleeping
- 3 – high chance of dozing or sleeping

These situations include when:

- sitting and reading
- watching TV

- sitting inactive in a public place
- travelling as a passenger in a car for more than an hour
- lying down in the afternoon
- sitting and talking to someone
- sitting after lunch (no alcohol)
- stopping for a few minutes while driving, e.g. at traffic lights

If you add up the scores, the total you get is the patient's Epworth Score.

If the Epworth Score is greater than 10, the patient may also suffer from OSA.

They may also be given:

- a medical examination
- a nasoendoscopy
- an overnight sleep study

Some children and teenagers snore.

This is often the result of:

- mouth breathing
- large tonsils

By the end of the mixed dentition/early second dentition, when other facial structures relative to the tonsils have grown, their problem usually disappears.

However, for adults diagnosed with OSA and/or snoring their problem does not go away.

SOCIAL PROBLEMS

It has obvious detrimental effects.

These include:

- an adverse effect on their social life
- marital problems, from sleeping apart in separate rooms to sleeping on the couch and even to separation and divorce
- poor-quality sleep, which affects concentration, reaction times, ability to cope, etc.
- sleep deprivation and tiredness experienced by the patient and those around them, which affects social interaction, tolerance, moods, etc.
- depression in some patients
- repercussions on their job, if they need to hold a driving license
- daytime drowsiness, often while travelling or driving

- loss of vitality, more time spent sitting, lack of energy, too tired to join in or be enthusiastic
- social embarrassment, e.g. fellow hotel guests complaining
- problems during holidays with a partner (having to book two separate rooms)
- sleeping on aircraft, etc.

Symptoms can include:

- raised blood pressure
- strain on the heart
- difficulty in concentration, sometimes affecting memory
- dry mouths, aggravating gingival/gum conditions
- depression, never feeling on top of things
- loss of libido

These are areas which can have a major impact on people's daily lives.

WHAT CAUSES THE SNORING NOISE?

Snoring usually emanates as a noise in the back of the throat as a result of a turbulent air flow.

During sleep:

- the muscles of the face, mouth, tongue and neck relax
- there is narrowing of the breathing passages
- the tongue drops back encroaching on the airway space
- the soft palate 'flutters' causing a noise

Factors making the problem worse:

- being overweight, especially in men as they carry excess weight around their necks
- drinking alcohol, especially last thing at night
- going to sleep after a heavy meal
- taking muscle relaxants, e.g. sleeping medication
- anatomical features such as retrognathia (receding lower jaw)

WHAT ARE THE SOLUTIONS?

- try to reduce excess weight
- reduce the intake of alcohol
- exercise more

Self-prescribing and 'over-the-counter' remedies

There are a variety of remedies which are sold 'off the shelf'.
These include:

- nasal strip worn over the nose
- nasal sprays
- nasal drops
- nasal expanders
- herbal pillows
- humidifiers
- ready-made mandibular advancement devices
(These are commercial devices sold to wear in the mouth but because these are not made to fit the individual patient but 'one size fits all' they have limited results.)

These appliances have the advantage of being:

- easily available
- inexpensive

The appliances also have disadvantages such as:

- poor fitting
- having a limited length of use
- being bulky
- possible effect on the occlusion
- lack of perseverance in patients for wearing them

Continuous positive airway pressure masks (CPAP)

These are prescribed mainly for OSA patients from the specialist sleep clinic.
A continuous positive airway pressure (CPAP) mask can be tried. This consists of a mask which fits over the nose and air is supplied under pressure from a pump. While considered to be the gold standard treatment, it does have some disadvantages.
Some patients:

- find these bulky
- feel wearing the mask is a little claustrophobic
- find it causes them to wake up with a dry mouth
- dislike the pressure on their faces
- find the sound of the pump used to circulate the air pressure is noisy and keeps them, and possibly their partner awake

Custom-made mandibular advancement devices for the patient

The patient can have a device made especially for them.

The purpose of the device is to position the lower jaw forward. As the tongue is attached to the floor of the mouth this is also automatically brought forward.

By doing this, the airway at the back of the throat widens and the tongue does not tend to block it, so air can pass more easily. The flow of air when the patient is sleeping is improved and the noise reduces or disappears.

A number of appliances are available, ranging from the complex and expensive to the relatively basic and inexpensive to produce. They all work using the same principle.

These are variously known as:

- Mandibular advancement devices
- Mandibular advancement splints
- Mandibular repositioning splints
- Functional appliances (twin block) which postures the lower jaw forward
- Herbst appliances which use metal telescopic connectors
- Thermo-formed splints

At the 'top of the range' these appliances have base plates made from:

- chrome cobalt (a very strong light alloy metal)
- gold

These:

- are smaller
- are more closely fitting
- provide more room for the tongue

At the other end of the scale, the simplest of these devices is the thermo-formed splint.

These:

- look like a sportsman's mouth guard
- fit on the upper and lower teeth and position the lower jaw forwards
- are easy to wear
- have a central anterior opening to allow patients to breathe through their mouths if necessary
- are made of ethyl vinyl acetate (EVA)
- can be made relatively quickly in the laboratory
- are relatively inexpensive due to the materials used

In addition to referrals from doctors and dentists and specialist sleep study centres, orthodontists in hospitals also receive referrals from their colleagues:

- respiratory consultants
- ear, nose and throat consultants

who

- have medically assessed these OSA and snorer patients and wish them to have such a device
- have found their patient unable to tolerate a CPAP machine and are trying an alternative

In the dental surgery at the assessment appointment, care is taken to record the amount of mandibular protrusion the patient can comfortably tolerate and to check that the patient has free movement of the temporo-mandibular joints (TMJs)

They must also have an adequate number of teeth.

When making and following up a thermo-formed mandibular advancement device, three visits are needed and the patient is then referred back to their dentist or doctor with a report.

WHAT IS NEEDED

At the first appointment, the nurse needs to prepare:

- *patient's clinical notes*
- *upper and lower impression trays*
- *beading or ribbon wax to extend them if necessary*
- *alginate, bowl and spatula*
- *wax for squash bite and postured bite*
- *method of softening wax, blow torch, flame or hot water*
- *container of cold water for cooling the postured bite*
- *bowl in case of gagging reflex*
- *mouthwash and tissues*
- *impression disinfectant solution*
- *sealed plastic bag for transit*
- *laboratory instruction sheet*

NB: This device (Figure 22.1) is intended to hold the lower jaw forward, thereby preventing the tongue from falling back and obstructing the flow of air to the sleeping patient. Therefore, the second bite recording is taken with the lower jaw in this protruded position. Care will be taken when designing the appliance to leave a space between the upper and lower parts so that mouth breathers will be able to take air in.

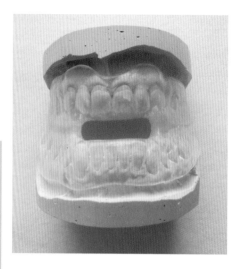

Figure 22.1 Mandibular advancement device.

THE PROCEDURE

The nurse needs to assist the clinician to:

- *ensure that the patient and staff are wearing personal protective equipment*
- *seat the patient comfortably in the chair, sitting upright for preference*
- *prepare wax bites, one single thickness, and the other 2–4 thicknesses, depending on the occlusion*
- *provide a bowl of cold water (after the postured bite is taken it must be taken out, cooled and re-inserted to check it is correct)*
- *make sure that the trays are well extended, use beading or ribbon wax*
- *mix upper and lower alginate impressions*
- the clinician takes the impression and records the bite
- *immerse the impressions and wax bites in disinfectant solution as per manufacturer's instructions*
- *fill in laboratory instruction sheet*
- *send both to the technician*

When the appliance has been made by the technician the patient returns for the second appointment to fit the device.

At the second appointment, the nurse needs:

- *to prepare patients, notes, with the Medical Devices certificate filed in them*
- *to prepare patient's model box*
- *to have the device ready*
- *a mouth mirror and ruler on a tray*
- *a suitable container for the patient to take home and use for storing the device when it is not in the mouth*

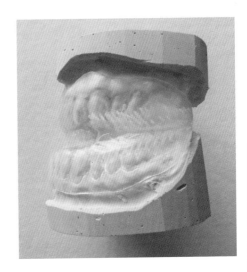

Figure 22.2 Lateral view of mandibular advancement device.

- *a hand mirror to show the patient the best method to insert and remove the device*
- *a patient instruction leaflet, giving instructions on cleaning, storage, etc.*

Then:

- *ensure that the patient and staff are wearing personal protective equipment*
- *seat the patient comfortably in the chair*
- the clinician fits the device
- *once the device (Figure 22.2) has been fitted, make sure that the patient:*
  - *can take it in and out themselves*
  - *knows how to clean it*
  - *is given written instructions*
  - *is supplied with a rigid box for storing it when not in use*

On the third appointment, the nurse needs to prepare only:

- *patient's clinical notes*
- *patient's model box*
- *mouth mirror*

The patient does not need to sit in the dental chair for this as this appointment is:

- to give feedback
- to assess any difficulties
- to quantify how successful it has been

If there has been adequate improvement, the patient continues to wear the device.

If there is no adequate improvement and the patient is not able or prepared to wear it, the device is discontinued. A letter is written to inform the referring doctor and their dentist that this is the case.

Further consideration regarding alternative options available to the patient will then have to be discussed. Surgery is an option to be considered when all the non-invasive methods have been tried and not been successful.

OUTCOME

Advantages:

- the success rate for these appliances is very good
- they are disinfected in a simple solution of Milton antiseptic
- they do not require a power supply to make them work
- as it is a non-invasive procedure, it is reversible
- when successful it has made a great improvement to the quality of life for OSA sufferers, snorers and for their families

Disadvantages:

- they do not last indefinitely
- they can become stained
- the joint between the upper and lower components can tend to split

Conclusion

Mandibular advancement devices can:

- reduce noise
- help to provide quality sleep
- reduce levels of tiredness
- benefit general health
- help the patients, self-esteem
- benefit relationships with partners

They are non-invasive:

- if successful, a good outcome
- they provide immediate relief for patients, their partners and those around them
- if unsuccessful, the patient has not been permanently affected by an irreversible process

Chapter 23

Model box storage and study models

At the beginning of every orthodontic patient's treatment, 'base line' records are taken to aid assessment, to monitor progress and for medico-legal purposes.

These include:

- study models
- radiographs
- intra-oral and extra-oral photographs

These should all be carefully stored as they contain confidential data which must be protected.

Study models are a very important part of the patient's treatment. They need to be available to the clinician at every appointment.

In order to produce them:

- Upper and lower alginate impressions are taken
- A wax squash bite is taken to record the occlusion

These are cast in the laboratory by the technicians using either a plaster or stone mix. Orthodontic models are trimmed in a specific way (Figure 23.1).

During the length of a course of treatment there can be several sets of impressions taken.

These can be for:

STUDY MODELS (Figure 23.2)

These are kept in the patient's model box, used for reference and as a record of the patient's occlusion at that time.

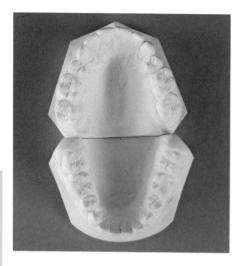

Figure 23.1 Example of the method of trimming orthodontic models.

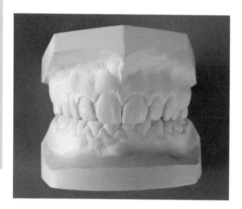

Figure 23.2 Study models.

STAGE MODELS

These are taken at the end of a stage of treatment, e.g. when a patient has completed the expansion stage of treatment and is going into fixed appliances.

WORK MODEL

The work model is the model on which the technician makes the appliance.

COORDINATION MODELS

When the pre-surgical orthodontic phase of treatment is completed, impressions are taken to confirm that the teeth have been moved into the planned position.

PLANNING MODELS

When the patient is to have orthognathic surgery, models are mounted on articulators. The models are cut and remounted to the planned occlusion to enable the surgeon to see the movement required at the operation. Also, to aid planning and assessment, e.g. for cases of hypodontia and some complex orthodontic cases, a Kesling set-up is done to prescription in the laboratory. This is a procedure whereby individual teeth are cut off a work model and re-set to the prescribed position to simulate future orthodontic tooth movements.

WAFER IMPRESSIONS

The models from these impressions are used to make the acrylic wafer that is used by the maxillo-facial surgeon in theatre during an osteotomy.

DEBONDING IMPRESSIONS

These are taken when the appliances are removed. The technician will cast two sets of models. One set is used as work models for making retainers and another as study models.

FINAL IMPRESSIONS

These are taken at the end of treatment, when the patient is discharged.

Many of these models must be kept as records. The initial and final models are a medico-legal record of:

- 'pre-treatment'

and

- 'post treatment'

MODEL BOX STORAGE AND STUDY MODELS

At the end of treatment, these models are PAR scored to measure the percentage of change that treatment has achieved.

PAR is an Occlusal Index and stands for *Peer Assessment Rating*.

When monitoring the percentage of improvement that has been achieved by orthodontic intervention, five areas are considered:

- anterior segments, upper and lower
- buccal occlusion, right and left
- overbite or open bite
- overjet
- centre line

Because the models for each patient need to be available at each visit, they must be stored in an easily accessible system.

There are many excellent systems and what works well for an individual surgery or unit is the best for them and the one they choose.

The system adopted is often governed by

- the number of patients under treatment, i.e. the number of boxes needed
- the size and accessibility of the storage area

The patient's individual box number can be stored:

- on their computer notes
- on their paper notes
- on a computer spreadsheet, e.g. MS Excel
- in an 'index of model boxes' book, kept in the model store room

One suggested method is:

- that boxes are filed in numerical order and cross referred in alphabetical order using an easily accessible racking or shelving system to maximise space and save time
- the number of each patient's box is written in their notes or fed into a computer with the patient's details

Given that there can be many hundreds of boxes in current use at any one time, a separate cross-reference book or spreadsheet is kept with details entered both ways:

- patient names listed alphabetically in the front of the book
- their number listed numerically in the back of the book

If one entry is overlooked, the other usually finds the models. It is a belt and braces method that works. If a patient's models are misfiled or incorrectly recorded, it takes a lot of time to find them!

MODEL BOX STORAGE AND STUDY MODELS

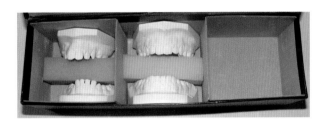

Figure 23.3 Models stored in box.

All the patient's details are noted:

- on a changeable label on the front of the box
- on the inside of the lid of the box, i.e.:
  - name
  - age
  - clinician

Names of patients must not be easily visible to other patients either in storage or in the surgery to comply with patient confidentiality and data protection.

All the patient's models should be boxed (Figure 23.3), before and after treatment and at other times if there has been more than one phase of treatment, e.g. a functional appliance before a fixed.

At the completion of treatment, when the patient is no longer under supervised retention, the patient's models are transferred from 'current' storage to the archive storage.

This can then:

- 'free' that number for another patient so the numbers will still run sequentially
- prevent that number becoming 'dead' and new patients having ever higher numbers

Due to the number of boxes stored in the 'dead' archive:

- they must be filed in alphabetical order
- in the year that their treatment was completed and they were discharged

This makes it easier to identify and dispose of models when they are no longer needed.

Orthodontic models are part of the patient's records and must be kept for 10 years post treatment, or until the patient is 25 years old.

All models have the patient's name and date when the impression was taken written on them.

Noting the patients' date of birth on the box is useful when calculating when the models can be discarded.

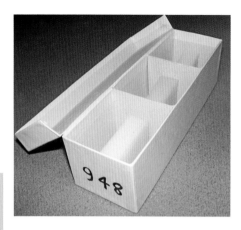

Figure 23.4 Model box.

It must be recorded in the patient's notes:

- if they have been moved from one storage site to another
- if they have been discarded

When discarding models, all traces of the patients' details must be obliterated from them before they are sent for crushing.

Patients who have had long or multi-disciplinary treatments often have more than one box.

Orthodontic storage boxes have three compartments, so they hold on average three sets of models (Figure 23.4). Some boxes have the upper and lower model stored apart; some have them stored together, with a foam pad kept between the teeth so that the occlusal surfaces of the teeth are not damaged.

When siting the 'dead' storage area it is as well to remember that the content of several hundred boxes weighs a ton!

Often, boxes for cleft patients or patients who underwent orthognathic surgery are marked with an additional coloured label. This is merely for fast identification and easier retrieval. Cleft lip and palate patients' boxes are also specially marked because their models must be kept for a longer period and records are taken at particular ages and intervals for National audit purposes.

Patients who have undergone surgery may also have a Max-Fax box stored as well.

In the future, digital models and three-dimensional images might overtake the plaster models but this technology in all surgeries may be some way ahead.

Chapter 24

Descriptions and photographs of most commonly used instruments and auxiliaries

Acid etch

Chemical gel used before primer to prepare tooth surface prior to bonding an attachment (Figure 24.1)

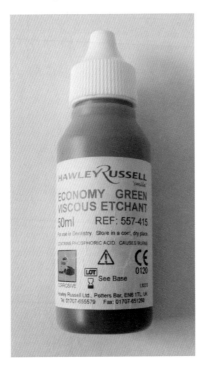

Figure 24.1

Adams clasp (crib)   Clasp (sometimes called a Crib) used on removable
appliances for retention (Figure 24.2)

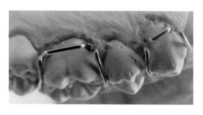

Figure 24.2

Adams pliers   Plier used to adjust wire components on removable
appliance (Figure 24.3)

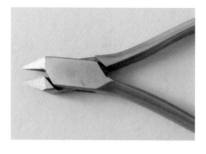

Figure 24.3

**Adhesive and
Primer**   Material that bonds brackets, tubes, etc. to teeth
(Figure 24.4)

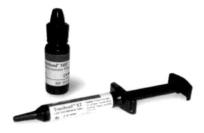

Figure 24.4

**Adhesive-removing
pliers**   Plier with a blade that removes adhesive from tooth
after debonding (Figure 24.5)

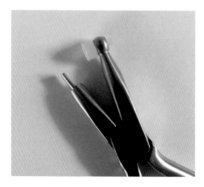

Figure 24.5

Aesthetic bracket   Less visible, non-metal bracket (Figure 24.6)

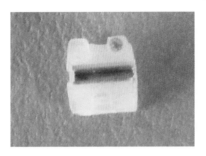

Figure 24.6

Appliance box   Box to keep removable appliance safe when out of the mouth, e.g. sport (Figure 24.7)

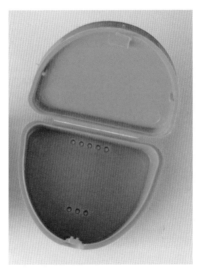

Figure 24.7

Arch wire   Formed wire used in fixed appliances (Figure 24.8)

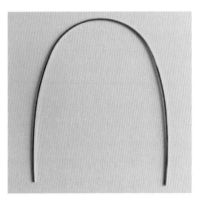

Figure 24.8

Arch wire stand   Convenient holder for many different sizes of arch wire (Figure 24.9)

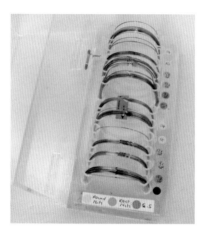

Figure 24.9

Australian wire   Type of spooled steel wire (Figure 24.10)

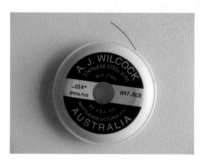

Figure 24.10

Band   Metal ring cemented around molar tooth (Figure 24.11)

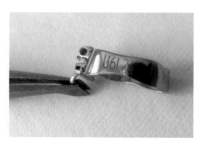

Figure 24.11

Band-slitter pliers   For cutting bands to release them from tooth (Figure 24.12)

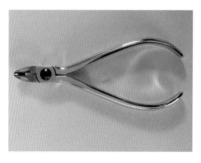

Figure 24.12

Bird-beak pliers   Multi-use with fixed appliances, popular, strong, has a round and a square beak (Figure 24.13)

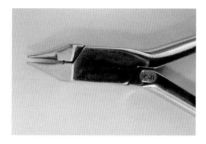

Figure 24.13

Bite stick   Nylon. Patient bites on this to fully seat metal band. Has triangular bite pad, which may be soft metal, autoclavable (Figure 24.14)

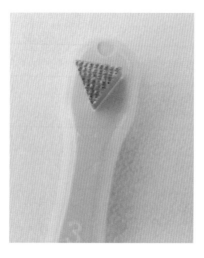

Figure 24.14

MOST COMMONLY USED
INSTRUMENTS AND AUXILIARIES

Bonded retainer   Wire or metal bar cemented to the lingual side of teeth as a fixed retainer (Figure 24.15)

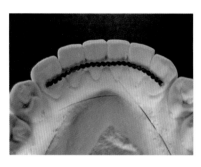

Figure 24.15

Bracket   A metal or ceramic attachment bonded to the teeth in fixed appliances through which the arch wire is slotted (Figure 24.16)

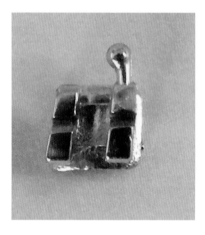

Figure 24.16

Bracket-holding tweezers   For use with direct bonding. Holds individual bracket, when placing onto tooth. Press handles together to open beak to release bracket (Figure 24.17)

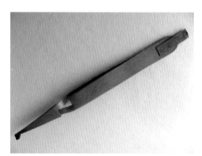

Figure 24.17

Bracket-removing pliers

For use on steel, plastic and ceramic brackets (Figure 24.18)

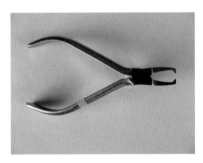

Figure 24.18

Braided wire

Wire made up of several strands braided together (Figure 24.19)

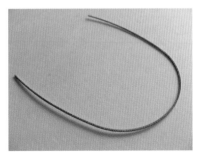

Figure 24.19

Buccal tube

Tube, can be bonded to the cheek surface of tooth or may be welded to a band. Tube can be of round or rectangular section into which the arch wire fits (Figure 24.20)

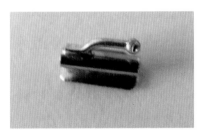

Figure 24.20

MOST COMMONLY USED
INSTRUMENTS AND AUXILIARIES

Bump-r-sleeve   Clear sleeving, fits over arch wire to prevent wire cutting into soft tissues (Figure 24.21)

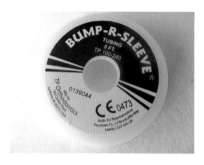

Figure 24.21

Cement   Lining material inside the band when fitted on a tooth, eliminates space between band and enamel (Figure 24.22)

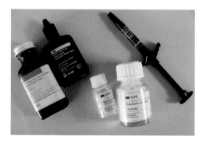

Figure 24.22

Chain   Line of joined elastic links, available in various sizes, can be clear or coloured (Figure 24.23)

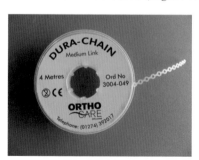

Figure 24.23

Cheek retractor   Plastic frame, keeps lips and cheeks away from teeth and gives better vision, access and moisture control (Figure 24.24)

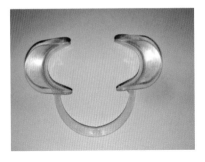

Figure 24.24

Cleat   Metal attachment that can be welded to bands or bonded to teeth (Figure 24.25)

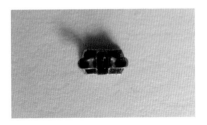

Figure 24.25

Coil (open and closed)   Sold on spools, to either open or maintain a space (Figure 24.26)

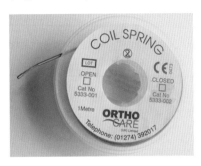

Figure 24.26

Coil springs (NiTi)   Fits over fixed appliance attachment and used to close spaces, particularly of extraction sites (Figure 24.27)

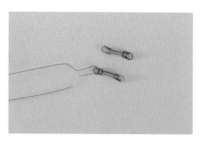

Figure 24.27

Coon's ligature-tying pliers   Plier for tying metal ligatures (Figure 24.28)

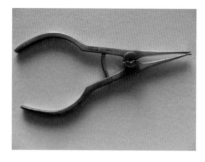

Figure 24.28

Curing light   Used to cure light activated adhesive and cement (Figure 24.29)

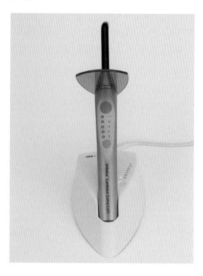

Figure 24.29

Dappen's pot   Container (often disposable) for use with etch, primer and prophy paste (Figure 24.30)

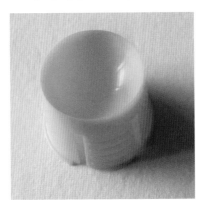

Figure 24.30

Debonding bur   Bur for removing composite at deband (Figure 24.31)

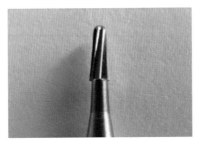

Figure 24.31

Director   Double ended hand instrument with notches to help hold wire when ligating (Figure 24.32)

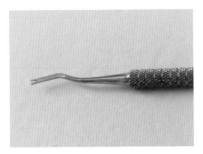

Figure 24.32

MOST COMMONLY USED
INSTRUMENTS AND AUXILIARIES

Distal-end cutters   Cuts arch wire flush or close to the distal end of the buccal tube. Holds the excess after cutting (Figure 24.33)

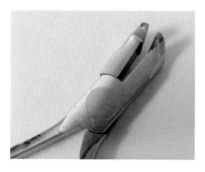

Figure 24.33

Dividers   Adjustable instrument for measuring distances between teeth (Figure 24.34)

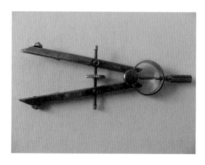

Figure 24.34

Elastic placer   For ease in attaching elastics (Figure 24.35)

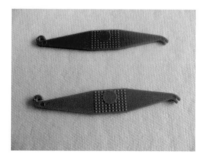

Figure 24.35

Elastomerics Rings to secure wires onto brackets, often known as O-rings (Figure 24.36)

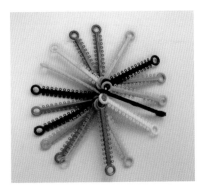

Figure 24.36

Essix retainer Removable retainer, fits over teeth, no metal clasps, cribs or bows (Figure 24.37)

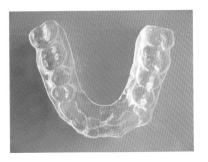

Figure 24.37

Eyelet Bondable or weldable metal attachment, used for attaching traction (Figure 24.38)

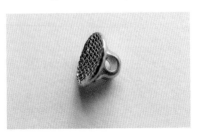

Figure 24.38

MOST COMMONLY USED
INSTRUMENTS AND AUXILIARIES

**Fixed lingual
retainer wire**

Wire especially for fixed retainers (Figure 24.39)

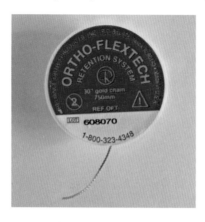

Figure 24.39

**Force module
separator**

Another name for Separating pliers (Figure 24.40)

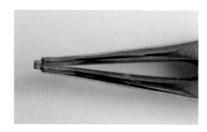

Figure 24.40

Hawley retainer

Removable retainer, acrylic baseplate with metal bow,
cribs and clasps (Figure 24.41)

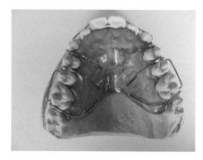

Figure 24.41

High pull head caps Readymade caps, to combine with EOT modules (Figure 24.42)

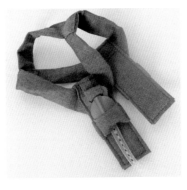

Figure 24.42

Intermaxilliary elastics Elastics that are fitted between upper and lower dental arches (Figure 24.43)

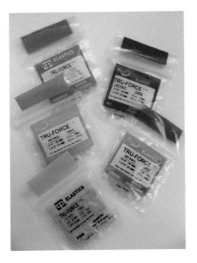

Figure 24.43

Interproximal stripper For reducing contact points between the teeth (Figure 24.44)

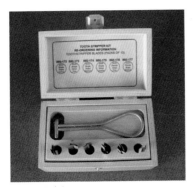

Figure 24.44

MOST COMMONLY USED
INSTRUMENTS AND AUXILIARIES

Interspace brush   Single tufted brush for cleaning around arch wire
                              (Figure 24.45)

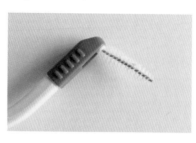

Figure 24.45

Kobyashi hook   Hook shaped end of ligature, used with inter maxillary
ligature   elastics (Figure 24.46)

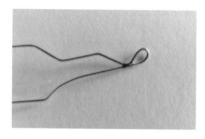

Figure 24.46

Ligature director   Double-ended hand instrument, notched to tuck in end
                              of ligature away from soft tissues (Figure 24.47)

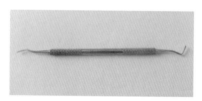

Figure 24.47

Light-wire pliers   Tapered beaks, one round, one square for bending
                              fixed appliance arch wires (Figure 24.48)

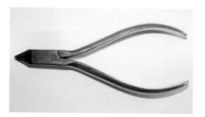

Figure 24.48

Lip bumper   Strips of rubber which fit over anterior brackets, useful for patients who play musical instruments by mouth (Figure 24.49)

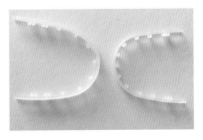

Figure 24.49

Lip retractor   Same function as cheek retractors (Figure 24.50)

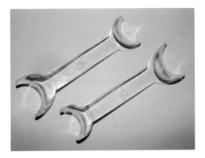

Figure 24.50

Mandibular advancement device   Appliance that postures the lower jaw forward to open the airway to reduce snoring noise (Figure 24.51)

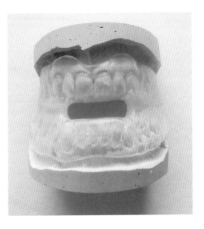

Figure 24.51

MOST COMMONLY USED
INSTRUMENTS AND AUXILIARIES

Mathieu haemostat   Used to ligate wires and hold elastomerics. Ratchet lock on closing, spring loaded, easy to turn in hand, firm grip (Figure 24.52)

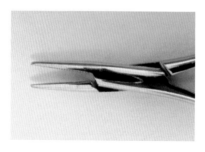

Figure 24.52

Mauns cutters   Heavy-duty plier, used to cut wire outside the mouth, e.g. face bows (Figure 24.53)

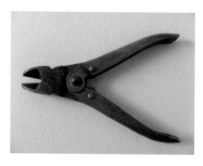

Figure 24.53

Mershon pusher   Used to seat and contour bands to teeth. Can have chunky, standard or round handle (Figure 24.54)

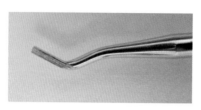

Figure 24.54

Microbrush   Disposable applicators (Figure 24.55)

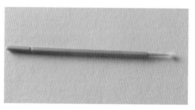

Figure 24.55

Mitchell trimmer   Double-ended multi-purpose hand instrument (Figure 24.56)

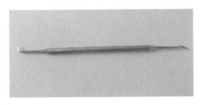

Figure 24.56

Model box   For storage of models for individual cases (Figure 24.57)

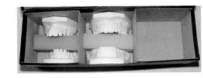

Figure 24.57

Mosquito forceps   Positive locking, to place elastomerics, ligatures, etc., beaks smooth or serrated (Figure 24.58)

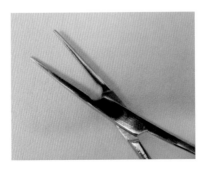

Figure 24.58

Occlusal registration bite recorders   To hold wax when recording a bite (Figure 24.59)

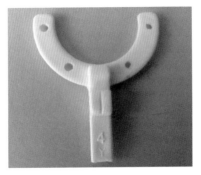

Figure 24.59

MOST COMMONLY USED
INSTRUMENTS AND AUXILIARIES

O-rings　　　　　　Name given to elastomerics (Figure 24.60)

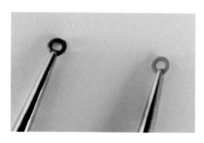

Figure 24.60

Par ruler　　　　　Ruler used to measure Indices (Figure 24.61)

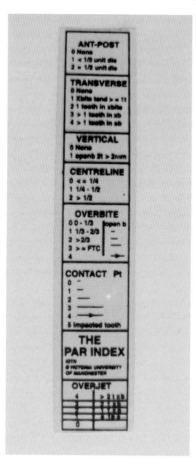

Figure 24.61

Photographic mirrors

Double-sided, chromium-coated glass, several shapes (Figure 24.62)

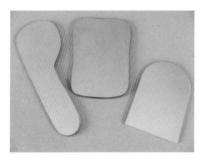

Figure 24.62

Pin and ligature cutting pliers

Cuts pins (Begg), ligatures and light wires up to 015″ (Figure 24.63)

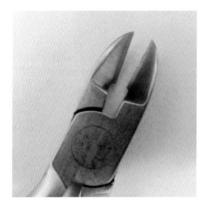

Figure 24.63

Posted arch wire

Arch wire that has posts attached to it, which point gingivally, used for traction (Figure 24.64)

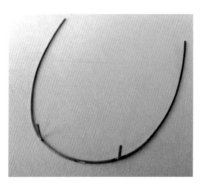

Figure 24.64

Posterior band Has pad, rests on occlusal surface to ease the band off
removing pliers the tooth, replacement heads available (Figure 24.65)

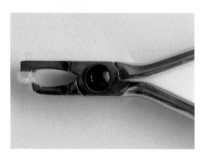

Figure 24.65

Primer Solution applied to teeth, after etchant before adhesive
during bonding procedures (Figure 24.66)

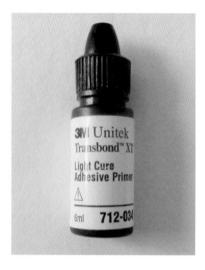

Figure 24.66

Retainer brite Kills germs, helps control calculus and keeps removable
appliances clean and fresh (Figure 24.67)

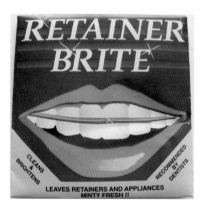

Figure 24.67

Retainer case   For keeping retainers safe when not in mouth (Figure 24.68)

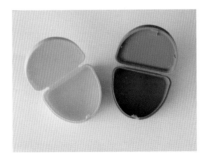

Figure 24.68

Reverse curve wire   Pre-formed arch wire used to help reduce deep overbite (Figure 24.69)

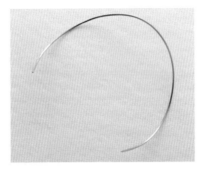

Figure 24.69

Rotation wedge   Auxiliary in fixed appliance therapy (Figure 24.70)

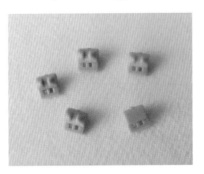

Figure 24.70

Ruler   Chrome or stainless steel, 6″ (150 mm) (Figure 24.71)

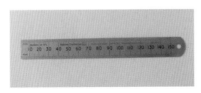

Figure 24.71

MOST COMMONLY USED
INSTRUMENTS AND AUXILIARIES

Safety face bows   For use with headgear (Figure 24.72)

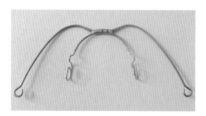

Figure 24.72

Safety glasses   Orange – for use with curing lights (Figure 24.73); tinted – for general use (Figure 24.74)

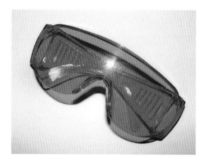

Figure 24.73

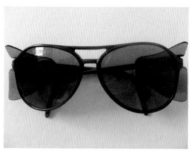

Figure 24.74

Safety swivel key   Key for turning expansion screws (Figure 24.75)

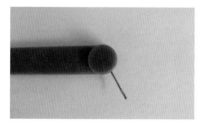

Figure 24.75

Self-etch primer   Single-use application of self-etch primer, used when bonding attachments to teeth (Figure 24.76)

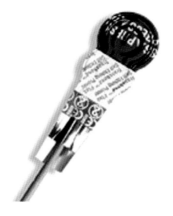

Figure 24.76

Separating pliers   For placing separators and elastics (Figure 24.77)

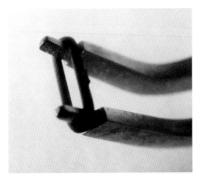

Figure 24.77

Silicone (medical grade)   To protect soft tissues from irritation by fixed appliance (Figure 24.78)

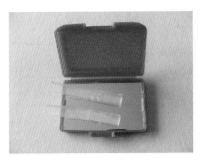

Figure 24.78

Southend clasp   Metal attachment, used on upper centrals on removable appliances (Figure 24.79)

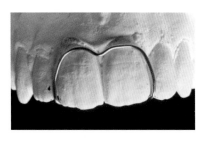

Figure 24.79

Temporary anchorage device   Mini implant to provide anchor point (Figure 24.80)

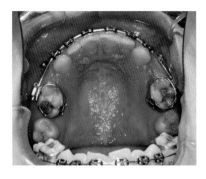

Figure 24.80

Tweed rectangular arch bending pliers   Wire-bending pliers, for use on square and rectangular wire; use two together (Figure 24.81)

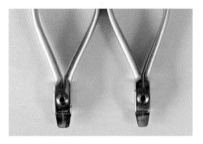

Figure 24.81

Twirl-on   Brand name of hand instrument used for inserting elastomerics (O-rings) (Figure 24.82)

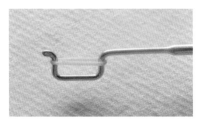

Figure 24.82

Weingart utility pliers	Serrated pads, tapering beaks, can also be angled (Figure 24.83)

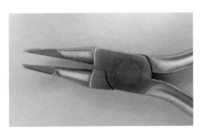

Figure 24.83

Z spring	Spring used in removable appliances (Figure 24.84)

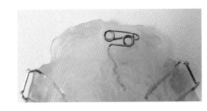

Figure 24.84

Zing string	Elastic thread used to provide traction (Figure 24.85)

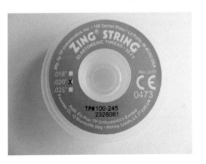

Figure 24.85

MOST COMMONLY USED
INSTRUMENTS AND AUXILIARIES

ACKNOWLEDGEMENT

Figures 24.4, 24.22, 24.29, 24.66 and 24.76 are reproduced with permission of 3M Unitek. © 2010 3M Unitek. All rights reserved.

Chapter 25

Certificate in Orthodontic Nursing and extended duties

In addition to the initial National Certificate and NVQ Course and Examination, a variety of post-registration qualifications are available. Additional qualifications are currently being developed to meet the needs of the profession and career pathways for dental nurses. Nurses who work in the field of orthodontics are very fortunate to have a post-registration qualification in their specialty and the orthodontic profession was very supportive of its development.

WHAT IS IT?

The Certificate in Orthodontic Nursing was introduced in 2001 and is now well established as a popular post-registration qualification, with the National Examination Board for Dental Nurses (NEBDN) as its awarding body. Responsibility for registering students for this award lies with the training centres.

WHO QUALIFIES TO GO ON THE COURSE?

It is a course intended for dental nurses who work within orthodontics. Nurses who want to go on to gain this Certificate must:

- be registered with the General Dental Council
- have the support of their employer

THE FEE STRUCTURE FOR THE COURSE

The cost of the course varies between training centres. There is a registration and examination fee payable to NEBDN.

Up-to-the-minute information on this, and where the training centres are located, is available either by contacting the National Examining Board for Dental Nurses (NEBDN) or by looking on the internet.

WHAT DOES THE COURSE CONTAIN?

Once on the course, nurses will need to attend lectures and instruction on the theoretical aspect of the qualification. For this there is a comprehensive syllabus.

They also need to show that they can apply this knowledge in a practical setting. For this they need to compile a Record of Experience which records their competencies.

The written **Examination Paper** consists of two parts:

- Paper A, which is made up of multiple choice questions
- Paper B, which consists of short answers to structured questions

The examination is taken at the nurses' own training centre and is independently assessed by NEBDN examiners.

The **Record** of **Experience** has three parts.

Part 1: Log Sheets

Students must record their involvement in the treating of at least 50 cases. Of these:

- 10 must be in removable appliance therapy, including 5 patients with functional appliances
- 10 patients in fixed appliance therapy

Part 2: Case Studies

The student must produce two detailed case studies. These must be:

- to advise a patient on oral hygiene and instruction on how to look after their orthodontic appliance
- to follow a patient whose orthodontic treatment was part of an interdisciplinary interface

Part 3: Evidence of Competence

The student will be expected to demonstrate competence in relation to:

- taking of clinical photographs/slides
- completion of cephalometric tracing, digitisation and measurement
- assisting with the taking and handling of impressions
- casting of study models
- contributing to the fitting and adjustment of orthodontic appliances

THE SYLLABUS FOR THE CERTIFICATE IN ORTHODONTIC NURSING

SECTION ONE   ANATOMICAL STRUCTURES RELATIVE TO ORTHODONTICS
1.1   Define the function and structure of the:
    1.1.1   muscles of mastication
    1.1.2   muscles of facial expression and soft tissues
    1.1.3   tongue
    1.1.4   maxilla and mandible
1.2   Describe the:
    1.2.1   structure and morphology of deciduous teeth and their eruption dates
    1.2.2   structure and morphology of permanent teeth and their eruption dates
    1.2.3   growth and development of the mandible and maxilla
    1.2.4   basic principles of the biology of teeth movement

SECTION TWO   CLASSIFICATION OF MALOCCLUSION
2.1   Describe and identify:
    2.1.1   skeletal classification
    2.1.2   incisor
    2.1.3   molar
    2.1.4   define diagnostic terms, e.g. overbite, crossbite

SECTION THREE   ORTHODONTIC TREATMENT
3.1   understand the aims and limitations of orthodontic treatment
3.2   understand the risks and benefits of orthodontic treatment
3.3   explain how treatment progress is monitored
3.4   discuss finishing and detailing techniques
3.5   explain the function, need and duration of retention

SECTION FOUR   ORTHODONTIC RECORDS
4.1   Describe:
    4.1.1   the importance of orthodontic record taking
    4.1.2   the use of written assessment records and medical history
    4.1.3   effective methods of clinical photography
    4.1.4   the types of radiographs and their relevance in orthodontic treatment
    4.1.5   an effective system for the storage of orthodontic models
4.2   Demonstrate:
    4.2.1   effective methods of clinical photography
    4.2.2   completion of cephalometric tracing, digitising and measurement
    4.2.3   the chairside procedure for the production of study models

SECTION FIVE   ORTHODONTIC APPLIANCES

5.1   Active and passive removable appliances:

    5.1.1   explain the indications

    5.1.2   describe the advantages and disadvantages

    5.1.3   describe the components of an appliance

    5.1.4   describe the construction of an appliance

    5.1.5   describe the different types and uses of appliances

    5.1.6   describe the chairside procedures required to produce a working model

    5.1.7   identify the instruments and equipment used during the construction of appliances and describe and demonstrate their use during the procedure

    5.1.8   identify the materials used during the procedure and demonstrate their use

    5.1.9   explain the nature of the advice given to patients on the care of appliances

    5.1.10   be able to identify the level of damages to appliances and their potential for repair

5.2   Fixed appliances:

    5.2.1   explain the indications

    5.2.2   describe the advantages and disadvantages

    5.2.3   describe the different types and uses of appliances

    5.2.4   describe the components of an appliance and the importance of brackets and bands

    5.2.5   describe the construction of an appliance

    5.2.6   describe the chairside procedures required to construct appliances

    5.2.7   demonstrate the orientation of brackets

    5.2.8   describe the faults which can occur when positioning brackets and their effects

    5.2.9   describe and define the types and use of orthodontic wire

    5.2.10   describe the use of intra-oral elastics and other auxiliaries

    5.2.11   identify the instruments and equipment used during the construction of appliances and describe and demonstrate their use during the procedure

    5.2.12   identify the materials used during the procedure and demonstrate their use

    5.2.13   explain the nature of the advice given to patients on the care of appliances

5.3   Extra-oral traction:

    5.3.1   describe the principles of use and directional force

    5.3.2   identify the components of extra-oral traction

    5.3.3   identify types and describe the fitting of safety headgear

CERTIFICATE IN ORTHODONTIC NURSING AND EXTENDED DUTIES

11.3 Describe how the practice of orthodontics is regulated and how these regulations affect the orthodontic dental nurse and other members of the orthodontic team

11.4 Explain what is meant by the term 'informed consent'

SECTION TWELVE ORTHODONTIC INDICES AND CLINICAL GOVERNANCE

12.1 Demonstrate the use of the Index of Orthodontic Treatment Need (IOTN)

12.2 Demonstrate the use of the Peer Assessment Rating (PAR)

12.3 Understand the relevance of prioritising treatment

12.4 Describe and be able to use methods of assessing outcomes of treatment

12.5 Understand the complexity of treatment and the hierarchy of treatment provider

The Syllabus for the Certificate in Orthodontic Nursing is reproduced by kind permission of the NEBDN.

For many orthodontic nurses, the Certificate in Orthodontic Nursing is a logical progression in their career pathway. For some, it is a means to an end, for others it is a gateway to their next step, to become an Orthodontic Therapist. Please see Chapter 26.

In addition to the Certificate of Orthodontic Nursing, other courses run for post-registration qualifications include:

- Certificate in Oral Health Education
- Certificate in Dental Sedation Nursing
- Certificate in Special Care Dental Nursing
- Certificate in Dental Radiography

More nurses are now attending the PAR Occlusal Indices courses.

CERTIFICATE IN ORTHODONTIC NURSING AND EXTENDED DUTIES

MODULE IN THE TAKING OF DENTAL IMPRESSIONS

This module is only available through Orthodontic Training Centres accredited by NEBDN. Candidates will be required to attend a programme of theoretical instruction and also compile evidence of practical competence through a Record of Experience. In order to qualify for the award, a dental nurse must:

- hold the Certificate in Orthodontic Nursing qualification or currently be registered on an orthodontic course
- be registered with the General Dental Council
- have the support of their employer

WHAT DOES THE COURSE CONTAIN?

Learning outcomes

- Clinical procedures involved in the taking of dental impressions
- Communication within the dental environment
- Legislation and Safety Guidelines controlling the taking of impressions

Record of experience

The Record of Experience assesses the application of knowledge and the skills required in practical situations.

It must be completed and forwarded to NEBDN by the Training Centre 4 weeks before the examination is taken.

Log sheets

Candidates must complete 25 log sheets, at least 5 of which must be for an adult patient, detailing their involvement in the taking of impressions.

Examination

The Training Centre undertakes internal assessment of the Record of Experience. The final external moderation and verification is undertaken by NEBDN.

Underpinning knowledge and understanding are assessed by an examination which candidates are able to undertake within their own Training Centre on the second Friday of June or December. The 30-minute examination consists of 25 multiple-choice questions.

Certification

In order to be awarded a certificate for the module, a candidate must:

- complete the Record of Experience

and

- achieve a pass standard in the multiple choice question paper

Certificates will be awarded to successful candidates.

ACKNOWLEDGEMENT

This information is reproduced by kind permission of NEBDN and is subject to change without notice.

Chapter 26

Orthodontic therapists

For the orthodontic dental nurse who has taken the Certificate of Orthodontic on Orthodontic Dental Nursing and wants to expand their ongoing professional development further, the next logical step may be to apply to enrol on a course to become an orthodontic therapist.

The orthodontic therapy courses began in 2007 and there was a lot of interest in them from the beginning.

While some of the training is given at the training centres, each student will work under the supervision of their own trainer. The trainers have themselves been trained to undertake this. They will be a specialist orthodontist who works in either secondary care, such as a hospital department or a community clinic, or in primary care in a specialist practice.

Courses follow a modular format.

At the start of the course, the first 8 weeks will contain the core teaching.

The first week they are based at their training base.

The following week they are in their own training unit, training practice.

This pattern continues over eight weeks.

In this way the student has undergone four 5-day weeks of training.

So the 20 days of core training are completed.

The successful candidate has to be able to have sufficient free time to attend the core teaching.

Competition for places is keen. Applications are taken from:

- dental nurses
- dental hygienists
- dental therapists
- dental technicians

All need to be registered with the General Dental Council (GDC) and have experience of working full time (or the equivalent) for at least a year post qualification.

Dental technicians training is different, so they have to be able to show that they have been on a foundation course to be able to understand the clinical and management side of working with patients in a dental surgery. They must also be able to show knowledge of cross infection, etc.

The orthodontic therapist works under the prescription of a dentist. Only the dentist can:

- decide on a treatment plan
- make a diagnosis of disease
- adjust or activate an arch wire

THE SYLLABUS FOR ORTHODONTIC THERAPY

Biomedical sciences and oral biology

- Have the knowledge and understanding of those aspects of the biomedical sciences, oral physiology and craniofacial, oral and dental anatomy that are significant in the management of patients
- Be familiar with those aspects of general anatomy, physiology and biochemistry relevant to orthodontic therapy

Medical emergencies

- Be competent at carrying out resuscitation techniques
- Have knowledge of how to identify medical emergencies and provide immediate management of anaphylactic reaction, hypoglycemia, upper respiratory obstruction, cardiac arrest, fits, vasovagal attack, inhalation or ingestion of foreign bodies or haemorrhage
- Be familiar with the principles of first aid

Dental biomaterials science

- Be competent at the correct selection and manipulation of the dental biomaterials used by the orthodontic therapists
- Have knowledge of the science that underpins the dental biomaterials used by the orthodontic therapist
- Have knowledge of the limitations of such dental biomaterials
- Be familiar with those aspects of biomaterials safety that relate to the work of the orthodontic therapist

Pain and anxiety control

- Be competent at managing fear and anxiety with behavioural techniques and empathise with patients in stressful situations
- Be familiar with the manifestations of anxiety and pain, and the various methods available for their management control

ORTHODONTIC THERAPISTS

Human disease

- Have knowledge of the scientific principles of sterilisation, disinfection and antisepsis
- Be familiar with the implications of a positive medical history and the main medical disorders that may affect the provision of orthodontic treatment
- Health and safety and infection control
- Be competent at implementing and performing satisfactory infection control and preventing physical, chemical and microbiological contamination in the clinic and the laboratory
- Be competent at arranging and using the working clinical and laboratory environment in the most safe and efficient manner
- Have knowledge of health and safety legislation as it affects clinical and laboratory practice

Comprehensive oral care

- Be competent at working with other members of the dental team
- Be competent at interpreting and working to, an orthodontic care plan or prescription
- Have knowledge of the role of the orthodontic therapist within the framework of the dental team
- Have knowledge of when to refer the patient to a dentist, where treatment is beyond the training or experience of the orthodontic therapist
- Be familiar with the organisation of the orthodontic services within the United Kingdom

Behavioural sciences, communication skills and health informatics

- Be competent at using the latest information technology
- Be competent at communication with patients, their families and carers, other members of the dental team and other healthcare professionals
- Have knowledge of managing patients from different social and ethnic backgrounds
- Have knowledge of working as part of the dental team
- Be familiar with the social and psychological issues relevant to the care of patients

Law, ethics and professionalism

- Be competent at maintaining full accurate clinical records
- Have knowledge of responsibilities of consent, duty of care and confidentiality

ORTHODONTIC THERAPISTS

- Have knowledge of patients' rights and how to handle complaints
- Have knowledge of the range of skills of other members of the dental team
- Have knowledge of the regulatory functions of the GDC
- Have knowledge of their responsibilities in relation to the referral of patients
- Be familiar with the legal and ethical obligations of registered members of the dental team
- Be familiar with the obligation to practice in the best interests of the patient at all times
- Be familiar with the need for lifelong learning and professional development
- Be familiar with the law as it applies to records

CLINICAL ORTHODONTICS

Clinical records

- Be competent at taking intra-oral and extra-oral photographs of patients, and photographs of models and radiographs
- Be competent at taking dental impressions
- Be competent at taking and checking occlusal records, including gnathological face bow readings
- Be competent at casting, basing and trimming orthodontic models
- Be competent at producing a cephalometric analysis of a skull radiograph by contemporary methods

Principles of orthodontics

- Have knowledge of the features of normal and ideal occlusion
- Have knowledge of the classification of malocclusion
- Have knowledge of the principles of tooth movement, force application and anchorage
- Have knowledge of common orthodontic appliance systems and their mechanical principles
- Be familiar with the aetiology of malocclusion
- Be familiar with the limitations of orthodontic treatment
- Be familiar with the potential risks and benefits of orthodontic treatment, including iatrogenic damage

Orthodontic instruments

- Be competent at identifying and selecting appropriate instruments for the task to be carried out
- Be competent at using equipment and instruments safely

ORTHODONTIC THERAPISTS

- Be competent at maintaining instruments
- Removable appliance placement
- Be competent at inserting passive removable appliances
- Be competent at inserting active removable appliances previously adjusted by a dentist
- Be competent at fitting orthodontic headgear
- Be competent at fitting orthodontic face bows having been previously adjusted by a dentist
- Be competent at measuring elastic headgear forces

Fixed appliance placement

- Be competent at placing and removing orthodontic separators
- Be competent at identifying and selecting orthodontic bands appropriate for the patient
- Be competent at placing, adapting and cementing bands to achieve an ideal fit
- Be competent at identifying attachments appropriate for individual teeth
- Be competent at cleaning and preparing the tooth surface for orthodontic bonding
- Be competent at using orthodontic adhesives and cements
- Be competent at placing attachments, including bonded retainers, onto the teeth in the correct position
- Be competent at preparing arch wires
- Be competent at inserting and ligating arch wires and arch wire auxiliaries
- Be competent at ligating groups of teeth together
- Be familiar with the technique of welding attachments to bands

Fixed appliance removal

- Be competent at releasing and removing ligatures
- Be competent at removing arch wires and arch wire auxiliaries
- Be competent at removing cemented and bonded attachments
- Be competent at differentiating between dental tissues, dental deposits and cement residues from the teeth
- Be competent at supragingival cleaning and polishing of the teeth using both powered and manual instrumentation, and at stain removal and prophylaxis where directly relevant to orthodontic treatment

Orthodontic emergency care

- Be competent at identifying damaged and distorted orthodontic appliances
- Be competent at taking limited action to relieve pain and make an appliance safe in the absence of a dentist

ORTHODONTIC THERAPISTS

- Be competent at identifying when a situation is beyond the orthodontic therapist's expertise and requires the patient to be seen by a dentist
- Have knowledge of the need to arrange early attention by a dentist following the emergency treatment

In the future this list could be extended still further to include:

- taking out sutures on the instruction of a dentist
- apply topical fluoride varnish as indicated by the dentist
- repair the acrylic components on removable orthodontic appliances
- measure and record gingival indices and plaque indices

However there are some procedures that are reserved for:

- dentists
- dental therapists
- dental hygienists

These include:

- giving local anaesthetics
- doing deep (sub gingival) scaling
- fitting temporary dressings
- re-cementing crowns or bridges

ACKNOWLEDGEMENT

The Syllabus is reproduced by kind permission of the General Dental Council.

Chapter 27

Professional groups for orthodontic dental nurses

THE ORTHODONTIC NATIONAL GROUP FOR DENTAL NURSES AND THERAPISTS

The ONG was formed as an independent specialist group for Dental Nurses in the UK and Ireland in June 1994. From their initial meeting their aims and objectives were clear.

AIMS

- *to act on behalf of all dental nurses and to advance high standards by developing the orthodontic nurses' role*

OBJECTIVES

- to develop the orthodontic dental nurses' (and now also therapists') role within the orthodontic specialty
- to provide Continuing Professional Development through Study Days, the Journal, the Nurses Day programme at British Orthodontic Conference and two Dental Nurse Competitions
- to liaise with all professional bodies, including the British Orthodontic Society, the British Dental Association, the General Dental Council, the Royal Colleges and the Deaneries
- to manage the Group's finances, business plan and strategies so that these objectives are realised

From the onset, their goal was to create career pathways for dental nurses, which would provide them with ongoing professional development, extended duties and recognition as Dental Care Professionals (DCPs).

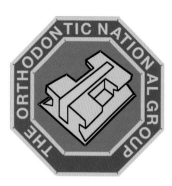

Figure 27.1 The ONG logo. (Reproduced with the kind permission of the Orthodontic National Group.)

The Group has a distinctive badge and logo consisting of an orthodontic bracket (Figure 27.1).

The bracket has a yellow line filling the bracket slot which recognises the affiliation with dental nursing.

In 2005, the title of the Group name was amended to 'Orthodontic Nurses and Therapists' to encompass these rapidly developing roles as Dental Care Professionals.

A prime objective was always to develop the orthodontic dental nurses' and therapists' role within the specialists group. The curriculum for the Orthodontic Therapy course had input from the ONG and it was due in part to their direct representation to the GDC, that the title Orthodontic Therapist was accepted.

ONG were also represented on the group that worked on the Curriculum for the now well-established post qualification Certificate in Orthodontic Nursing.

In order to achieve this, the Group has always maintained a small and efficient elected Committee. All of them are busy working orthodontic nurses, so are able to relate to issues and difficulties facing their colleagues. They are professional nurses working on behalf of professional nurses.

STRUCTURE OF THE GROUP

The Committee meets every quarter and has its Annual General Meeting at the British Orthodontic Conference which is usually held in September. In recent years, in addition to the Committee, the posts of Chief Executive Officer and, more latterly, that of President have been added. The Group has been represented at the General Dental Council, the British Dental Association and the Royal Colleges.

EDUCATION

ONG has aimed to provide a focus for orthodontic education and development. As part of the British Orthodontic Conference, the nurses have a parallel programme of two sessions. The ONG have been invited by the BOS to submit suggested topics and speakers for this. This Nurses Day proves very popular and there are often some welcome visitors as, if space allows, a good number of orthodontists sit in on lectures in the auditorium. Sometimes, there is not enough room to accommodate them as each year the number of nurse delegates tops 400 making it significantly the largest meeting of orthodontic nurses in the country.

As part of the Nurses Day, there are two competitions. The Orthodontic Nurses Prize is sponsored by TOC and is awarded for the best folder of work presented. It is always well subscribed and keenly fought, with many, many hours of work on display. There are cash prizes and a certificate for the winner, runner-up and third place.

The other competition, The Orthodontic Nurse of the Year, sees nurses giving a live 10-minute presentation to the audience. While the presentations are being given, there is rarely a seat to be had. Again, the standard is always high and competition keen. This is sponsored by 3M Unitek, again, for cash prizes and certificates. When the BOC was held in Paris in 2005, this competition, begun by ONG, was open to delegates from all over the world. Judges from Australia, Romania, Portugal and Canada listened to the presentations of nurses from New Zealand, Germany, the USA, Belgium, France, Ireland, Italy and the UK, with the UK lifting the first World Dental Nurse of the Year title. There is now such a competition in many countries; the idea took on an international dimension.

The ONG aims to organise two Study Days each year, held in different parts of the country. These are always well attended and while having a high educational content are good social occasions as dental nurses meet and greet.

Annual registration with the GDC for dental nurses now carries with it an expectation that they will maintain their level of CPD points, of 150 hours, spread over a 5-year period. Of these, 100 will be non-verifiable and 50 verifiable, of which medical emergencies must have at least 10 hours, disinfection and cross infection must have 5 hours and radiology and radiation also 5 hours. Other areas include, complaints handling, legal and ethical issues. All Study Days and Nurses Day at Conference carry verifiable CPD points.

JOURNAL

From the outset in 1994, the Group published a quarterly newsletter for its members, as part of their commitment to education. These have a strong bias towards clinical topics, with a high educational content to provide a source of Continuing Professional Development for its readers. There are also articles written for and by dental nurses which aim to keep members abreast of current policies, technical data and recent changes to legislation. The format and name of the newsletter changed in 2003 to become the Orthodontic National Group Journal.

LINKS WITH THE BRITISH ORTHODONTIC SOCIETY (BOS)

In 1997, the ONG became an affiliated organisation of the BOS who had for many years been encouraging the team approach within the specialty. Many orthodontists actively encourage their nurses to go on courses, to Conference, provide them with CPD and financially support their development. The BOS not only encourages the Nurses Day but also allows nurses access to the lectures on the Scientific Programme held in the main auditorium on other days. Throughout the year, they also welcome and encourage nurses to attend some of the meetings of the many groups that make up the Society.

THE FUTURE

ONG continues to liaise on behalf of its members with the orthodontic and wider dental community. It values professionalism, both from itself and its members. It is not just in the field of orthodontics that nurses benefit, as ONG continues to focus on assistance and guidance for their members across a wide variety of areas.

The contact details are:

The Orthodontic National Group for Dental Nurses and Therapists
12 Bridewell Place
London EC4V 6AP
UK
Tel.: 020 7353 8680
Website: www.orthodontic-ong.org

BRITISH ASSOCIATION OF DENTAL NURSES (BADN)

In addition to being an association which cares for the development of dental nurses and nursing in general in the UK, BADN has sub-groups which cater for dental specialties. There is one for orthodontic nurses, called the National Orthodontic Group (NOG) which members of the BADN can access, with full details of events in the BADN Journal.

The contact details are:

British Association of Dental Nurses (BADN)
PO Box 4
Room 200
Hillhouse International Business Centre
Thornton Cleveleys FY5 4QD
UK
Tel.: 0870 211 014
Website: www.badn.org.uk

PROFESSIONAL GROUPS FOR
ORTHODONTIC DENTAL NURSES

Useful contacts

British Orthodontic Society (BOS)

12 Bridewell Place
London EC4V 6AP
Email: ann.wright@bos.org.uk
Phone: 020 7353 8680
Fax: 020 7353 8682
Website: www.bos.org.uk

General Dental Council (GDC)

37 Wimpole Street
London W1G 8DQ
Email: dcp@gdc-uk.org
Tel.: 020 7887 3800
Fax: 020 7224 3294
Website: www.gdc-uk.org

British Dental Association (BDA)

64 Wimpole Street
London W1G 8YS
Email: enquiries@bda.org
Tel.: 020 7935 0875
Fax: 020 7487 5232
Website: www.bda.org

Orthodontic National Group for Dental Nurses and Therapists (ONG)

12 Bridewell Place
London EC4V 6AP
Email: ann.wright@bos.org.uk
Tel.: 020 7353 8680
Website: www.orthodontic-ong.org

British Association of Dental Nurses (BADN)

PO Box 4
Room 200
Hillhouse International Business Centre
Thornton Cleveleys
Lancashire FY5 4QD
Email: editor@badn.org.uk
Tel.: 01253 338360
Website: www.badn.org.uk

National Examining Board for Dental Nurses (NEBDN)

108-110 London Street
Fleetwood
Lancashire FY7 6EU
Email: info@nebdn.org
Tel.: 01253 778417
Fax: 01253 777268
Website: www.nebn.org

Companies supplying orthodontic equipment and sundries

American Orthodontics
Riverside House
2a Mill Road
Marlow SL7 1PX
Email: ortho@americanorthodontics.co.uk
Tel.: 01628 477921
Fax: 01628 477923
Website: www.americanortho.com

DB Orthodontics
Ryefield Way
Silsden BD21 4WT
Email: sales@dbortho.com
Tel.: 0800 7833552
Fax: 0800 7833363
Website: www.dbortho.com

Forestadent
21 Carters Lane
Kiln Farm
Milton Keynes MK11 3HL
E mail: richard@forestadent.co.uk
Tel.: 01908 568922
Fax: 01908 560611
Website: www.forestadent.co.uk

Hawley Russell Ltd
Station Close
Potters Bar EN6 1TL
Email: john@hawleyrussell.com
Tel.: 01707 655579
Fax: 01707 651268
Website: www.hawleyrussell.com

3M Unitek
3M House
Morley Street
Loughborough LE11 1EP
Email: 3MUnitek@mmm.com
Tel.: 01509 613305
Fax: 01509 613172
Website: www.3MUnitek.com

Ortho-Care (UK) Ltd
5 Oxford Place
Bradford BD3 0EF
E mail: Richardg@orthocare.co.uk
            kelvin@orthocare.co.uk
Tel.: 01274 392017
Fax: 01274 734446
Website: www.orthocare.co.uk

Precision Orthodontics Ltd
Ashley House
58-60 Ashley Road
Hampton TW12 2HU
E mail: post@precisionorthodontics.com
Tel.: 0208 979 9493
Fax: 0208 979 9478
Website: www.precisionorthodontics.com

The Dental Directory
6 Perry Way
Witham CM8 3SX
Email: sales@dental-directory.co.uk
Tel.: 01376 391291
Fax: 01376 500581
Website: www.dental-directory.co.uk

TOC
The Old Church
Collins Street
Avonmouth Village
Bristol BS11 9JJ
Email: info@tocdental.com
Tel.: 0117 975 5533
Fax: 0117 975 5575
Website: www.tocdental.com

Torque Orthodontics Ltd
PO Box 209
Shipley BD17 5WS
Tel.: 01274 581058
Fax: 0870 0516394
Email: sales@torqueorthodontics.com
Website: www.torqueorthodontics.com

T P Orthodontics
Fountain Court
12 Bruntcliffe Way
Morley
Leeds LS27 0JG
Email: tpeng@tportho.com
Tel.: 0113 2539192
Fax: 0113 2539193
Website: www.tportho.com

Optident Ltd
International Development Centre
Valley Drive
Ilkley LS29 8PD
Tel.: 01943 605050

Fax: 01943 604422
Email: sales@optident.co.uk
Website: www.optident.co.uk

This is merely a guide to some of the many companies that specialise in orthodontic equipment and supplies.

Glossary of terms

Abfraction – wear caused by tooth being too high on the bite

Abrasion – wear caused by repeated action, i.e. excessive tooth brushing

Aesthetic component – part of the Index of Orthodontic Treatment Need, relates to degree of malocclusion judged by appearance

Aesthetic plane – line used in tracing lateral cephalometric radiographs, from the soft tissue tip of the nose to the soft tissue tip of the chin

Alginate – a type of material used in taking orthodontic impressions

Aligner – clear plastic splints, which are worn to align teeth; several used in a course of treatment

Alveolar bone graft – addition of bone when it is lacking, e.g. cleft and implant patients

Alveolar ridge – part of mouth that carries the teeth

Anchorage – point from which force is applied

Angle's classification – a classification of malocclusion based on the relationship between the upper and lower first molars

Ankylosis – condition where the root is fused to the bone (often as a result of trauma); it is an anatomical fusion between the alveolar bone and the cementum and cannot be moved orthodontically

Anodontia – absence of teeth

Anterior – at the front of the mouth, opposite of posterior

Anterior open bite – where there is no contact when front teeth bite together

Anti-habit appliances – a fixed or removable appliance with wire built-in, which acts as deterrent to thumb or finger sucking

Apical – relating to the apex (tip) of the tooth root

Arch wire – wire which fits into the attached component of fixed appliance

Assessment – an orthodontic examination of a patient's malocclusion

Attrition – tooth wear caused by repeated tooth-on-tooth friction, e.g. bruxism (grinding of teeth, especially at night)

Ball end clasp – part of a removable appliance fitting into tooth undercuts to aid retention of the appliance

Banding – fitting molar bands

Begg retainer – upper acrylic retainer with labial bow but no Adams cribs

Bimaxillary – both maxilla and mandible

Bite-raising appliance – appliance with acrylic over the occlusal surfaces to disengage the occlusion

Bonded retainer – wire permanently fixed to teeth to stop them moving (nearly always lingual surface)

Bonding – fixing attachments directly to the tooth surface (brackets, cleats, etc.)

Bone harvesting – taking bone from one part of the body for use elsewhere

Brace – a commonly used term for an orthodontic appliance

Bruxism – grinding together of teeth, often in sleep

Buccal – relating to the cheek-facing surface of the tooth

Buccal segment – the first premolar to the last molar in a quadrant

Buccal sulcus – space between the teeth and alveolar bone and the cheek

Caries – dental decay

Casting – making a model of the teeth from an impression

Centre line – vertical line running between the upper and the lower central incisors

Centric occlusion – the occlusion of the teeth when they fully touch together from an open mouth position without displacing

Cephalometric analysis – results of measurements made on a cephalometric radiograph either using manual tracing or computer software

Cephalometric radiograph – a true side view radiograph of the skull and face showing the relationship between the teeth and relative facial bones

Cervical strap – strap used with extra-oral traction which is placed around the back of the neck, similar function to a head cap

Cheek retractor – plastic device to keep the lips and cheeks from coming into contact with the teeth

Cingulum pad – part of the palatal aspect of upper incisor crown, towards the cervical

Clasp – a wire used on a removable appliance to give retention

Class I – an occlusion which is normal but with tooth irregularities

Class II – a malocclusion where the upper teeth are forward in relation to the lowers; there are two divisions of this class

Class III – a malocclusion where the lower incisor teeth bite either edge-to-edge or in front of the upper incisor teeth

Cleats – a hook-shaped attachment which can be bonded to teeth or welded to bands

Cleft lip – where there is a congenital gap or notch in the upper lip/alveolus

Cleft palate – where there has been incomplete midline fusion of the palate before birth

Clinical crown – the part of the crown that is visible, e.g. that can be used for orthodontic attachments as opposed to the anatomical crown

Coil – can be supplied open or closed, usually comes on spools, hollow coiled wire which is put over an arch wire to either push open a space or prevent a space from closing

Congenital defect – one present before birth

Consultation – appointment between patient and orthodontist to assess and to discuss treatment options

Crossbite – where the lower teeth are incorrectly biting outside the upper teeth; can be applicable to buccal segment (posterior) or anterior teeth

Crowding – not enough space in the dental arch to accommodate the teeth in good alignment

Curing light – an ultra-violet light used to 'set' dental adhesives and cements

Debanding – removal of bands

Debonding – removal of brackets

Decalcification – loss of hard (mineralised) dental tissue through acid attack

Deciduous dentition – first teeth, which are lost, also called primary, milk or baby teeth; 20 in total, early loss of these can affect eruption and positioning of permanent teeth

Decontamination – cleaning of instruments prior to sterilisation

Dens-in-dente – a malformation; literally, a 'tooth within a tooth'

Dental age – the apparent age of the dentition, which may not be the same as the chronological age of the patient

Dental arch – the position and form of the teeth in the upper and the lower jaws

Dental health component – part of the Index of Orthodontic Treatment Need, deals with obvious clinical problems, such as crossbites, overjets, rotations, etc.

Deviation – when the mandible deflects in its path of closure

Diastema – gap between teeth, commonly upper central incisors

Digit sucking – thumb or finger sucking habit

Displacement – when the mandible's path of closure is deviated because there is an occlusal obstruction initially

Distraction osteogenesis – the lengthening of bones by a rapid expansion system following surgical cuts in the bone

Ectopic canine – a canine tooth that has been deflected from its natural path of eruption and has gone off course

Enamel – mineralised hard outer surface of the anatomical crown of both deciduous and permanent teeth

Erosion – where there is damage to the tooth from acid attack, especially 'sugar-free' and carbonated drinks

Eruption pattern – the timing of the eruption of deciduous and permanent teeth

Essix retainer – clear vacuum-formed, thermoplastic retainer, which looks like a thin gum shield and is usually worn at night

Expansion screws – screws which are turned to open and expand

Extra-oral – not in the mouth

Extra-oral anchorage – use of the back of the head or neck as anchor points

Facebow – an inner and outer bow welded together, used in extra-oral traction; the inner bow fits into the buccal tubes on a removable or fixed appliance

Fixed appliance – an appliance that is fixed to the teeth and cannot be removed by the patient

Fixed retainer – a retainer that is fixed to the teeth and cannot be removed by the patient

Fluoride – an element found naturally in water which impedes caries; often added to water supply, toothpaste and mouthwash

Frankfort plane – used in assessment and when tracing lateral cephalometric radiographs; a horizontal plane which is reckoned to be parallel with the ground when humans walk upright

Frenectomy – removal of the frenum

Frenum – web of fleshy tissue in both maxilla and mandible notably in the midline between the lips and the gingivae

Functional appliance – type of appliance, removable or fixed, that helps to reduce increased overjets and encourages better development of the mandible

Genioplasty – surgical repositioning of the chin

Gingiva – the gum around a tooth

Gingivitis – inflammation of the gums, which can be localised and may be chronic or acute

Growth spurt – a child's period of rapid growth, usually during puberty; helpful when using functional appliances

Hawley retainer – removable retainer made of acrylic and wire components

Headgear – consists of a cervical or head band and a facebow which fits onto either fixed tubes on bands or a removable appliance in the mouth

Hypodontia – congenitally missing tooth or teeth

Hypoplastic – poorly formed, e.g. enamel defects

ICON (Index of Complexity, Outcome and Need) – an assessment index measuring the severity of malocclusion and treatment complexity

Impaction – when the normal process of tooth eruption has not occurred because there is a resistance to it, e.g. wisdom tooth impacted into second molars

Impression – imprint, using a soft material that sets; when cast it gives a reproduction; alginate is most commonly used in orthodontics

Incisor relationship – how the upper and lower incisors relate in occlusion

Index of Orthodontic Treatment Need (IOTN) – index used for standardising the criteria of orthodontic need

Infra-occlusion – tooth or teeth at a lower level than the occlusal plane

Intermaxillary traction – tooth movement occasioned by force from a point in the opposing dental arch

Interproximal reduction – making space between the contact points of teeth using a fine bur, disc or blade to reduce the thickness of proximal enamel

Intramaxillary traction – tooth movement occasioned by force from a point in the same dental arch

Intra-oral – inside the mouth

Intrusion – moving teeth orthodontically into the alveolar bone

Invagination – an abnormal indentation in the crown of a tooth

Kesling set-up – from a cast of the teeth, individual plaster teeth are cut off and repositioned on the model, to a prescription

Labial bow – a wire bow over the 'front' of the anterior teeth

Labial segment – incisor teeth (often includes the canines)

Leaflets – information about treatment and care

Ligature – soft wire, e.g. used to tie in arch wires

Lingual arch – a metal wire formed to the lingual outline of the lower arch

Lingual arch wires – of various alloys, designed for use in lingual technique

Lingual orthodontics – treatment where the brackets are fixed onto the inside surface of the teeth

Lip line – the position of the upper lip outline in relation to the upper incisor teeth

Lip trap – when the lower lip gets trapped behind the upper front teeth

Macrodont – larger than normal tooth

Malocclusion – where there is an incorrect relationship between the dental arches and/or the teeth

Mandible – the lower jaw

Mandibular plane – used in tracing lateral cephalometric radiographs; line of the lower border of the mandible

Masel safety strap – strap which is placed over the external J hooks on a face bow to give extra security

Maxilla – the upper jaw

Maxillary plane – used in tracing lateral cephalometric radiographs, a line between the posterior and anterior borders of the hard palate

Mesiodens – a supernumerary tooth in the midline between the upper incisors

Microdont – smaller than normal tooth

Microdontia – abnormally small teeth

Midline

    Dental – upper and lower dental arches

    Facial – vertical line of face

Mini screws – temporary anchorage devices (TADs)

Model box – where patient's models are stored; each patient has their own individual box

Molar relationship – relationship mesiodistally of the occlusion of the first molars

Mouth guard – semi-flexible appliance worn to protect teeth when playing contact sports

Nickel titanium – alloy material from which some arch wires are made

O-ring – elastomeric module placed around a bracket to hold the archwire in slot, come in variety of colours

Obstructive sleep apnoea – condition where patient has incomplete sleep pattern, can sometimes be woken by feelings of not breathing and choking

Occlusal plane – used when tracing lateral cephalometric radiographs; a line between the teeth in occlusion

Occlusal rest – a wire component of a removable appliance which lies over the occlusal surface of a molar

Occlusion – the relation in contact between the upper and lower dental arches

Odontome – abnormal mass of dental tissue

Oligodontia – several congenitally missing teeth

Open bite – when opposing teeth are not biting together in occlusion

Oral hygiene – maintaining a clean and healthy mouth

Oral surgery – surgery relating to the mouth, both skeletal and dental, and soft tissue

Orthodontist – one who practices orthodontics; usually speciality trained and registered

Orthognathic surgery – surgery to the jaw(s) to correct malrelationship

Orthopantomogram (OPT) – radiograph taken as scan view of all the teeth; X-ray tube moves around the patient's head

Osteogenesis – see distraction osteogenesis

Osteotomy – surgical procedure to correct skeletal related malocclusion

Overbite – when the upper front teeth overlap the lower teeth vertically

Overjet – how much the upper front teeth protrude or retrude horizontally in relation to the lower teeth

Palatal arch – wire that spans the palate, soldered to bands cemented to the molars

Palate – roof of the mouth, there is a hard and a soft palate with the soft posterior to the hard

PAR – Peer Assessment Review; an occlusal index to measure on study models, the degree of improvement after orthodontic treatment

Peg-shaped – misshapen, usually conical, tooth crown

Periodontal – relating to the supporting tissues of the teeth

Permanent dentition – the adult quota of 32 teeth: 8 incisors, 4 canines, 8 premolars and 12 molars

Photographic mirrors – palatal, buccal or lingual mirrors for intra-oral photography

Piercing – oral jewellery, lip, cheek and tongue studs, or hoops

Plaque – a soft clear substance formed from saliva and bacteria

Porcelain primer – used on porcelain crown and veneers before attaching brackets

Positioners – removable 'retaining' appliances that are also actively moving certain teeth

Posterior – at the back, opposite of anterior

Posterior open bite – where teeth do not bite together towards the back of the mouth

Posturing habit – bringing the lower jaw forwards in order to close the lips

Proclined – angled forwards

Quad helix – upper fixed appliance to widen arch; quad = 4, helix = circle

Radiograph – an image made using X-rays

Rapid maxillary expansion – appliance cemented onto teeth, with an expansion screw in palate, turned by patient

Referral – request from a dentist for a specialist consultation

Relapse – the occlusion returning to pretreatment irregularities

Removable appliance – an appliance that can be taken in and out of the mouth by the patient

Retainer – an inactive appliance that holds teeth in position to prevent relapse; can be removable or fixed

Retention – maintaining corrected teeth in their corrected positions

Retroclined – angled backwards

Reverse pull headgear – system which aims to bring the maxillary arch forward; used in Class III cases

Roberts retractor – active removable appliance with a sprung labial bow, which has high circles built into it

Root resorption – when the root becomes shorter (sometimes occurs as a side effect of orthodontic treatment; can also be pathological)

Rotation – when a tooth is twisted from the correct position

Scissor bite – when upper buccal segment teeth bite totally outside lowers

Screws – can be used for expansion; used as temporary anchorage devices (mini screws)

Self-ligating brackets – brackets with an 'arm' that can open and close over the wire slot; avoids need for O-rings and ligatures

Separating pliers – pliers used for placing separating rings, also known as force separating pliers

Separating springs – used when rubber-separating rings will not slip through contact points, inserted using Weingart or spring-forming pliers

Separators – devices placed between the teeth to open space prior to fitting bands

Sharps box – container for all used or unwanted metal, wires, bands, etc.

Skeletal pattern – maxilla and mandible relationship, usually in antero-posterior plane

Sleep apnoea – disruption of normal sleep rhythm, often accompanied by snoring and an interrupted breathing pattern

Southend clasp – a clasp used on removable appliances, positioned at the cervical margin of upper centrals

Space maintainer – appliance that keeps space open in a dental arch

Spacing – natural gaps between teeth in the same dental arch

Speech and language therapist (SALT) – therapist who helps with speech, which is often an issue for patients with clefts

Spider screws – type of temporary anchorage device

Springs – used in both removable and fixed appliances to move teeth

Stability – ability of teeth to remain in their corrected position after orthodontic treatment

Sterilisation – to make sterile

Stripping – removing enamel mesially and distally to provide space

Study models – casts used as records

Submerged – tooth sinking back below the occlusal level into the gum

Supernumerary tooth – an additional tooth, more than usual; sometimes remains unerupted

T spring – Spring used on removable appliances, shaped like the letter 'T'

Temporary anchorage device – small screws which can be placed directly into the alveolar bone for a short time and are easily removed; they provide an anchorage point

Temporo-mandibular joint – complex joint where the mandible opens and closes (the condyles can be felt moving by your ears when you open and close your mouth)

Tongue studs – studs piercing the tongue

Tongue thrust – an involuntary habit; a strong movement which can cause problems with positions of dental arches and speech

Tooth wear – results of tooth surface loss

Torque – a force to correct the inclination of teeth labio/buccolingually

Tracing – measurements from a lateral cephalometric tracing

Traction – tension, pulling

Transposition – when position of teeth is interchanged, an abnormality

Trauma – injury

Traumatic occlusion – occlusion that is causing self-damage

Treatment plan – choice of treatment based on assessment

Twin blocks – functional appliance consisting of upper and lower removable appliances

Ugly duckling stage – 'goofy', spaced teeth (mixed dentition) with teeth appearing to be too large for the face

Wafer – plastic occlusal guide used in osteotomy operations

Wafer impressions – impressions taken to make a wafer

Wax – material used to record the relationship between the upper and lower teeth, also to protect the soft tissues from being rubbed by a fixed appliance

Wisdom teeth – third molars

Work models – models on which appliances are made, not kept as study models

X-rays – needed to produce radiographs

Z spring – spring used on removable appliances to procline incisors

Index

Note: Page numbers tagged with italic "f" refer to figures

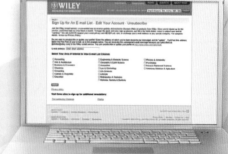
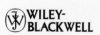